AF754954

Study Guide *for*

Gould's Pathophysiology *for the* Health Professions

Eighth Edition

Robert J. Hubert, BS
Laboratory Coordinator (retired)
Iowa State University
Department of Animal Sciences
Ames, Iowa

Andrew Sahawneh, BS, OD
Doctor of Optometry
University of South Alabama
Mobile, Alabama;
School of Optometry
University of Alabama at Birmingham
Birmingham, Alabama

Hannah Sahawneh, BS, OD
Doctor of Optometry
Iowa State University
Ames, Iowa;
School of Optometry
University of Alabama at Birmingham
Birmingham, Alabama

ELSEVIER

Elsevier
3251 Riverport Lane
St. Louis, Missouri 63043

STUDY GUIDE FOR GOULD'S PATHOPHYSIOLOGY FOR THE HEALTH PROFESSIONS, EIGHTH EDITION ISBN: 978-0-443-28427-4

Copyright © 2027 by Elsevier Inc. All rights are reserved, including those for text and data mining, AI training, and similar technologies.

For accessibility purposes, images in electronic versions of this book are accompanied by alt-text descriptions provided by Elsevier. For more information, see https://www.elsevier.com/about/accessibility.

Books and Journals published by Elsevier comply with applicable product safety requirements. For any product safety concerns or queries, please contact our authorized representative, Elsevier B.V., at productsafety@elsevier.com

Publisher's note: Elsevier takes a neutral position with respect to territorial disputes or jurisdictional claims in its published content, including in maps and institutional affiliations.

No part of this publication may be reproduced or transmitted in any form or by any means, electronic or mechanical, including photocopying, recording, or any information storage and retrieval system, without permission in writing from the publisher. Details on how to seek permission, further information about the Publisher's permissions policies and our arrangements with organizations such as the Copyright Clearance Center and the Copyright Licensing Agency, can be found at our website: www.elsevier.com/permissions.

This book and the individual contributions contained in it are protected under copyright by the Publisher (other than as may be noted herein).

Notice

Practitioners and researchers must always rely on their own experience and knowledge in evaluating and using any information, methods, compounds or experiments described herein. Because of rapid advances in the medical sciences, in particular, independent verification of diagnoses and drug dosages should be made. To the fullest extent of the law, no responsibility is assumed by Elsevier, authors, editors or contributors for any injury and/or damage to persons or property as a matter of products liability, negligence or otherwise, or from any use or operation of any methods, products, instructions, or ideas contained in the material herein.

Previous editions copyrighted 2023, 2018, 2014, 2011, 2006, 2002, and 1997.

Senior Content Strategist: Yvonne Alexopoulos/Kitchel Melissa
Senior Content Development Manager: Lisa P. Newton
Senior Content Development Specialist: Tina Kaemmerer
Publishing Services Manager: Deepthi Unni
Senior Project Manager: Nayagi Anandan
Design Direction: Brian Salisbury

Printed in India at Replika Press Pvt. Ltd.
Plot No. 310-311,
EPIP, HSIIDC, Kundli Industrial Park,
Sonipat, Haryana – 131028.

Last digit is the print number: 9 8 7 6 5 4 3 2 1

Working together to grow libraries in developing countries

ELSEVIER Book Aid International

www.elsevier.com • www.bookaid.org

Contents

1 Introduction to Pathophysiology

1. Describe the research stages necessary to demonstrate the safety and effectiveness of a new therapy.

2. Explain "off-label" use of a drug previously approved and give an example.

3. Briefly explain the impact of Artificial Intelligence in the health care arena.

4. Differentiate between an *acute* disease and a *chronic* disease.

5. What is the difference between an *epidemic* and a *pandemic*?

6. Cells adapt to environmental changes by changing their size, number, and type. For each of the following scenarios, identify the appropriate **adaptive cellular change** or changes that occur, using the following terms:

atrophy	metaplasia
hypertrophy	dysplasia
hyperplasia	neoplasia

i. a decrease in the size of a leg after being in a cast for 6 weeks:

ii. breast enlargement at puberty:

iii. a dramatic increase in muscle mass in an Olympic weightlifter:

iv. a very aggressively growing cancer mass:

v. a benign tumor growing along the spine:

vi. the changes that occur in the lower extremities of someone paralyzed below the waist:

vii. a pressure area under a poorly fitting denture:

viii. the changes that often occur over years in the respiratory tract of a smoker:

Copyright © 2027 by Elsevier, Inc. All rights are reserved, including those for text and data mining, AI training, and similar technologies.

ix. the changes responsible for an abnormal Pap smear:

x. the response of the skeletal system to excessive growth hormone:

xi. the thyroid gland's response to hypersecretion of thyroid-stimulating hormone:

xii. the liver's response to prolonged drug intoxication (e.g., chronic alcohol abuse):

xiii. the changes that occur in the gallbladder with the development of gallstones:

xiv. the thyroid gland's response to decreased iodine intake:

xv. the effect of decreased pituitary function on the adrenal glands:

xvi. the development of callus on the hands of an individual involved in heavy physical labor:

7. Which of the cellular adaptations above is considered the **most dangerous**? Explain why.

8. Explain the **significance** of anaplasia.

9. List eight causes of cellular damage.

i.

ii.

iii.

iv.

v.

vi.

vii.

viii.

Copyright © 2027 by Elsevier, Inc. All rights are reserved, including those for text and data mining, AI training, and similar technologies.

10. Complete the following crossword puzzle:

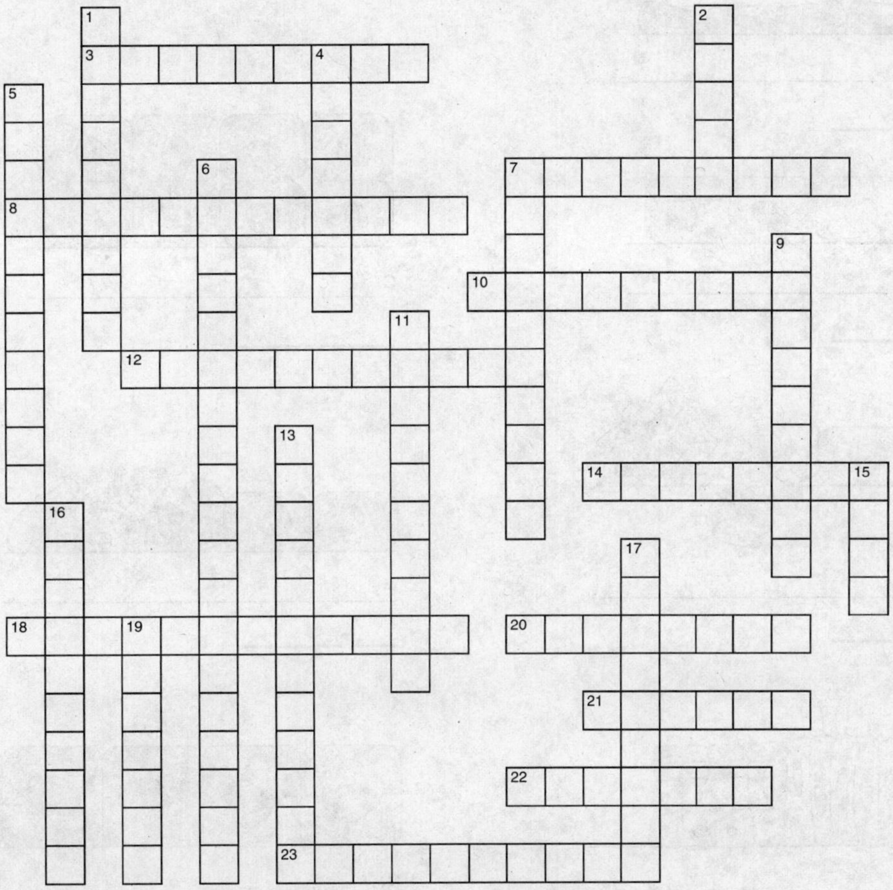

ACROSS

3. a tumor
7. number of new cases of a disease
8. worsening of a disease
10. death rate
12. issue enlargement caused by an increase in cell number
14. tissue death
18. development of a disease
20. the study of the cause of a disease
21. a specific local change in tissue
22. condition that continues for a prolonged period
23. originating inside the body

DOWN

1. condition in which cells fail to develop specialized features
2. condition with sudden onset and severe symptoms
4. subjective response to illness
5. tissue enlargement due to increased cell size
6. shoveling snow on a cold day (may cause heart problems)
7. unknown cause
9. condition resulting in atypical cervical cells
11. disease caused by a treatment procedure
13. contagious condition
15. objective indicator of a disease
16. substitution of one mature cell type with a different cell type
17. originating outside the body
19. decreased O_2

Copyright © 2027 by Elsevier, Inc. All rights are reserved, including those for text and data mining, AI training, and similar technologies.

11. Identify the following cellular adaptations:

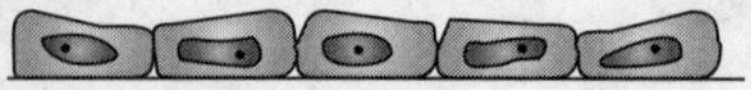

a. ____________________

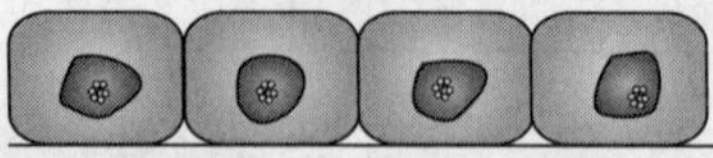

b. ____________________

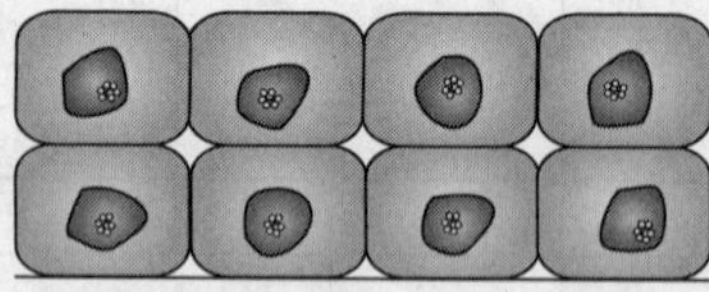

c. ____________________

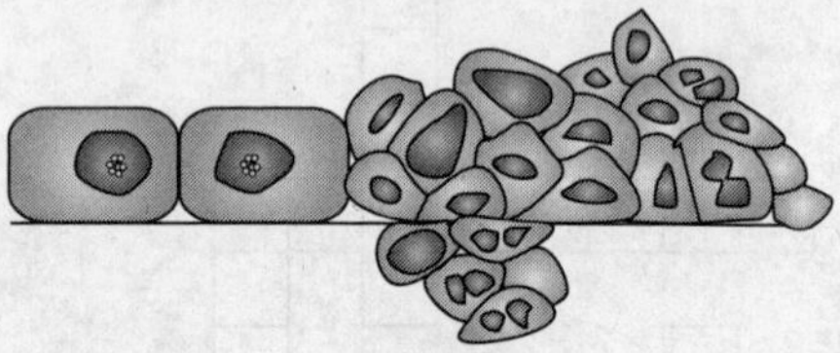

d. ____________________

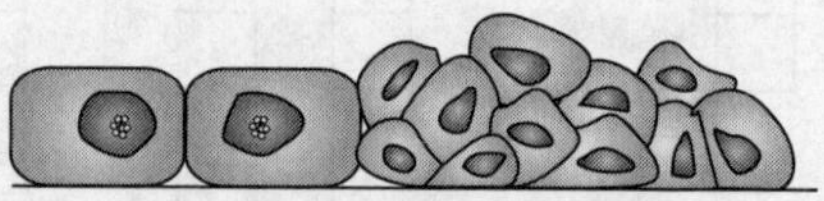

e. ____________________

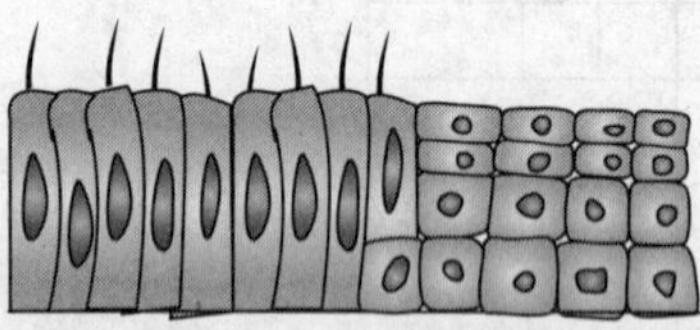

f. ____________________

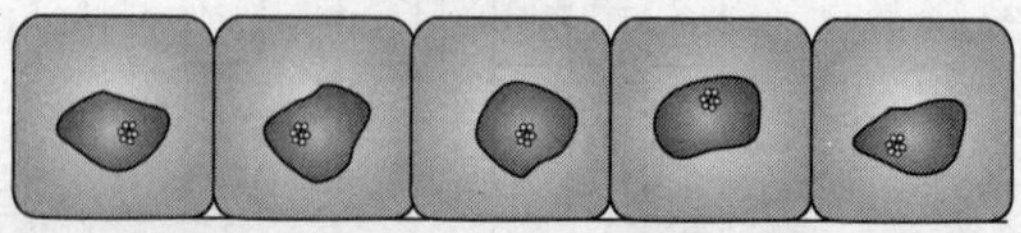

g. ____________________

Copyright © 2027 by Elsevier, Inc. All rights are reserved, including those for text and data mining, AI training, and similar technologies.

2 Fluid, Electrolyte, and Acid-Base Imbalances

EDEMA

1. Define **edema**.

2. Identify the four **general causes** of edema and explain how each one results in accumulation of fluid in the extracellular compartment.

3. For each of the following examples, state which of the causes identified in the previous question is responsible for edema formation:

   i. a swollen arm after mastectomy (surgical removal of a breast):

   ii. the abdominal swelling that accompanies liver failure:

   iii. the swelling that accompanies inflammation:

   iv. the generalized edema that occurs in severe kidney disease:

   v. swelling of the ankles that often happens at the end of the day or after prolonged standing:

   vi. swelling that occurs after multiple tooth extractions:

   vii. edema that may accompany cancer:

   viii. edema that accompanies burns:

   ix. edematous hands and ankles that sometimes accompany excessive ingestion of sodium:

   x. the abdominal swelling that occurs with starvation:

   xi. swelling of the ankles associated with heart problems:

   xii. swelling associated with allergic reactions, such as hives:

4. Identify at least eight **effects of edema**.

Copyright © 2027 by Elsevier, Inc. All rights are reserved,
including those for text and data mining, AI training, and similar technologies.

DEHYDRATION

5. List seven **causes** of dehydration.

6. Describe the **manifestations** of dehydration. What is the **most serious complication** of dehydration?

7. Identify the **compensatory mechanisms** that are recruited during dehydration.

8. Explain why an infant is more vulnerable than a young adult to fluid loss and dehydration.

9. Define **third-spacing** and provide examples of conditions where it occurs.

ELECTROLYTE IMBALANCES

10. Identify the **electrolyte imbalance** or imbalances that could develop in each of the following situations:

    i. renal failure:

    ii. prolonged vomiting:

    iii. insufficient secretion of antidiuretic hormone:

    iv. prolonged use of corticosteroids:

    v. hyperparathyroidism:

    vi. excessive sweating:

    vii. prolonged immobility:

    viii. diuretic therapy:

    ix. aldosterone insufficiency:

    x. inadequate dietary intake of vitamin D:

    xi. cancers involving bone:

    xii. prolonged diarrhea:

Copyright © 2027 by Elsevier, Inc. All rights are reserved,
including those for text and data mining, AI training, and similar technologies.

11. Define **tetany**. Identify the electrolyte imbalance in which tetany occurs.

12. Identify the electrolyte imbalances that affect normal **cardiac function**.

13. What electrolyte excess may result in the formation of **kidney stones**?

14. Explain how sodium imbalances affect nerve conduction and fluid shifts.

15. Describe how calcium balance is controlled in the body, including the roles of parathyroid hormone, calcitonin, and vitamin D.

ACID-BASE IMBALANCES

16. What is the pH range of normal human plasma? At what pH levels does death usually result?

17. Identify the three mechanisms that control or compensate for pH.

18. State the normal **bicarbonate ion to carbonic acid ratio** required to maintain normal serum pH.

19. Identify the **four major buffer systems**. Which is the major extracellular fluid buffer?

20. Explain how the respiratory system compensates for changes in serum carbon dioxide or hydrogen ion levels.

21. Explain how the renal system compensates for acid-base imbalances.

22. For each of the following scenarios, identify which acid-base imbalance could potentially develop. Also identify the compensatory mechanism(s) that might prevent this from occurring:

    i. chronic bronchitis:

    ii. induced vomiting (e.g., bulimia):

    iii. narcotic or barbiturate overdose resulting in respiratory depression:

    iv. extreme weight loss resulting in lipolysis:

    v. panic attack with hyperventilation:

Copyright © 2027 by Elsevier, Inc. All rights are reserved,
including those for text and data mining, AI training, and similar technologies.

vi. pneumonia, with severe bronchial congestion:

vii. chronic diarrhea:

viii. renal failure:

TREATMENT OF IMBALANCES

23. Describe the general principles for treating fluid, electrolyte, and acid-base imbalances.

Copyright © 2027 by Elsevier, Inc. All rights are reserved, including those for text and data mining, AI training, and similar technologies.

3 Introduction to Basic Pharmacology and Other Common Therapies

1. Once a drug is administered, the actual blood levels of this drug are dependent on several factors influencing the individual. What are some of these factors?

2. Describe the difference between **dose** and **dosage**.

3. Distinguish between the **therapeutic effects** and **adverse or side effects** of a drug.

4. Briefly describe some specific forms of adverse drug reactions that may affect your clients.

5. Medications may be administered by a number of different routes. Describe what is meant by each of the following drug routes, and state several examples of medications that are commonly taken this way:

   i. **topical**:

   ii. **transdermal**:

   iii. **oral**:

   iv. **sublingual**:

   v. **subcutaneous**:

   vi. **intramuscular**:

   vii. **intravenous**:

   viii. **inhalation**:

6. Drugs are used for both systemic and local effects. Which route of administration is used to achieve a **local effect**?

Copyright © 2027 by Elsevier, Inc. All rights are reserved,
including those for text and data mining, AI training, and similar technologies.

7. Complete the following chart comparing and contrasting various routes of drug administration:

	Onset of Action	Advantages	Disadvantages
Topical			
Transdermal			
Oral			
Sublingual			
Subcutaneous			
Intramuscular			
Intravenous			
Inhalation			

8. Arrange the routes of drug administration according to rapidity of onset, from the fastest to the slowest.

9. Describe what happens to a drug once it is absorbed into the blood.

10. Explain the manner in which many drugs exert their effects at a cellular level.

11. Where are most drugs **metabolized**? How is this achieved?

Copyright © 2027 by Elsevier, Inc. All rights are reserved, including those for text and data mining, AI training, and similar technologies.

12. How are most drugs or their metabolites **excreted** from the body?

13. Explain the ways in which liver or kidney disease could affect drug activity.

14. Why are individuals with chronic lung disease considered to be at high risk for complications when they receive a general anesthetic?

15. Explain how each of the following factors may influence drug action:

    i. age:

    ii. body weight:

    iii. sex:

    iv. psychological factors/emotional state:

    v. presence of disease (e.g., heart disease, liver disease, kidney disease):

    vi. time of administration (in relation to meals; time of day):

    vii. route of administration:

    viii. drug dosage:

    ix. drug formulation (e.g., liquid, capsule, enteric coated):

    x. client compliance:

    xi. environmental factors (e.g., temperature, odors, noise):

    xii. drug interactions:

16. Define the following terms, and state an example for each:

    i. hypersensitivity reaction:

    ii. idiosyncratic reaction:

Copyright © 2027 by Elsevier, Inc. All rights are reserved, including those for text and data mining, AI training, and similar technologies.

iii. potentiation:

iv. synergism:

v. antagonism:

vi. tolerance:

vii. placebo:

17. Differentiate between the **generic** and **chemical names** of a specific drug.

18. What are the five types of complementary therapies identified by the NIH?

19. Describe each of the following **treatment modalities**:

i. **physiotherapy:**

ii. **speech therapy:**

iii. **occupational therapy:**

iv. **homeopathy:**

v. **osteopathy:**

vi. **aromatherapy:**

vii. **chiropractic therapy:**

viii. **massage therapy:**

ix. **biofeedback:**

20. Explain the basis of Asian concepts of healing such as acupuncture, shiatsu, and yoga.

21. Which agency in the United States regulates the production, labeling, distribution, and other aspects of drug control?

Copyright © 2027 by Elsevier, Inc. All rights are reserved, including those for text and data mining, AI training, and similar technologies.

4 Pain

1. Provide a comprehensive list of factors that can initiate pain.

2. Differentiate between the origin of **somatic** and **visceral** pain.

3. Name three chemical compounds produced by the body that will stimulate pain receptors.

4. Outline the steps involved in the perception of pain, from the stimulus to interpretation. Include all the anatomical structures that are involved in the pathway.

5. Explain the mechanism by which endorphins can block pain impulses.

6. What is meant by **referred pain**? Explain how it occurs. Describe an example of referred pain.

7. Compare and contrast acute and chronic pain in terms of onset, duration, causes, and effects.

8. Outline measures used to control pain, including the rationale for each.

9. Identify conditions treated with trigger point injections and the substances typically injected.

10. Identify factors that may influence an individual's response to pain.

Copyright © 2027 by Elsevier, Inc. All rights are reserved,
including those for text and data mining, AI training, and similar technologies.

11. Complete the following chart, which compares and contrasts nonnarcotic and narcotic analgesics:

	Nonnarcotic Analgesics	Narcotic Analgesics
Action		
Adverse effects		
Uses		
Examples		

12. Identify three general types of anesthesia and state an example of how each would be employed.

13. Describe A delta and C fibers, comparing their structure and role in pain transmission.

14. Explain the gate-control theory of pain. How does this theory explain the modulation of pain signals, and what are some practical applications of this theory in pain management?

Copyright © 2027 by Elsevier, Inc. All rights are reserved, including those for text and data mining, AI training, and similar technologies.

5 Inflammation and Healing

1. What is the body's **first line of defense**?

2. Identify the body's **second and third lines of defense**.

3. Which of the three lines of defense are specific? Explain what is meant by "specific defense mechanism."

4. Define **phagocytosis**. Identify types of cells that are phagocytic.

5. What is **inflammation**, and what is its basic function? Identify some causes of inflammation.

6. Identify the two main events of the **"vascular response"** that occur during an inflammatory response. Explain their function as part of the response and the direct effects of each event.

7. Identify the **four cardinal signs** of an inflammatory response and the cause of each.

8. Outline the sequence of events involved in the **cellular response of inflammation**.

9. Match each of the following terms with the appropriate definition.

a. involved in cell-mediated immunity	i. neutrophils
b. elevated during allergic responses	ii. basophils
c. secrete histamine	iii. eosinophils
d. the first cells to migrate to an injured area	iv. macrophages
e. involved in antibody production	v. mast cells
f. elevated during chronic inflammations	vi. monocytes
g. a source of macrophages	vii. T lymphocytes
h. phagocytize microorganisms	viii. B lymphocytes

Copyright © 2027 by Elsevier, Inc. All rights are reserved,
including those for text and data mining, AI training, and similar technologies.

10. List the **systemic effects of inflammation**, and identify the reason that each of these manifestations occurs.

11. List some potential complications that may develop as a result of inflammation.

12. Compare and contrast **acute and chronic inflammation**, using the following chart:

Characteristic	Acute Inflammation	Chronic Inflammation
Causative agents		
Signs and symptoms		
Duration		
Cells involved		
Treatment		
Results		

13. What is the four-letter acronym that lists the approach to first aid for injury-related inflammations?

14. Identify the differences between **nonsteroidal antiinflammatory drugs (NSAIDs)** and **glucocorticoids or steroidal antiinflammatory drugs**.

15. Identify differences between **NSAIDs** and **acetaminophen**.

Copyright © 2027 by Elsevier, Inc. All rights reserved, including those for text and data mining, AI training, and similar technologies.

16. Identify additional **nonpharmacological therapies/treatment** that could be used to treat inflammation, particularly conditions that are chronic, such as arthritis.

17. Differentiate between the processes of **resolution and regeneration**.

18. Many factors influence **tissue healing**. Explain how the following factors could complicate or delay healing, stating at least one example to illustrate each one:

    i. nature of the tissue/location of the wound:

    ii. nutritional status of the injured individual:

    iii. condition of the wound:

    iv. drugs being taken:

    v. age of the individual:

    vi. presence of foreign material in the wound:

    vii. blood supply:

    viii. presence of infection:

    ix. degree of immobilization/irritation of the injured tissue:

    x. pre-existing disease/medical problems:

19. Identify potential complications that may occur during the healing process with scar formation.

20. Describe the four **classifications of burns** based on:

    i. depth of tissue damage:

    ii. body surface area involved:

21. Explain why full-thickness burns initially may be painless but later become very painful.

Copyright © 2027 by Elsevier, Inc. All rights are reserved,
including those for text and data mining, AI training, and similar technologies.

22. Other than tissue destruction, what are complications that may arise from a burn?

23. List some of the actions that may be taken to aid in the prevention of infection in the healing of a burn.

24. Fill in values on the diagram used to assess burn area using the rule of nines.

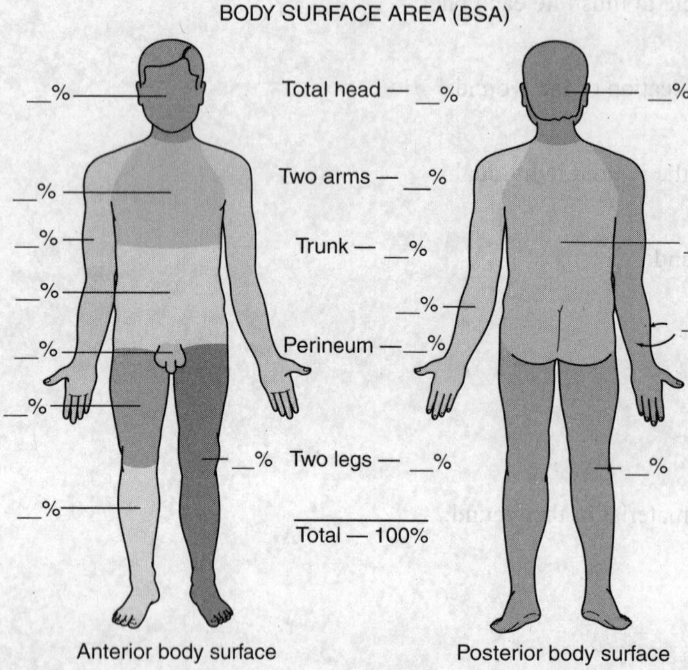

25. Explain the need for increased dietary intake of protein and carbohydrates during healing of a burn injury.

26. Some herbs and spices have powerful antiinflammatory properties. Name three of these herbs or spices and their possible use.

Copyright © 2027 by Elsevier, Inc. All rights are reserved, including those for text and data mining, AI training, and similar technologies.

6 Infection

1. Describe how a bacterium's environmental requirements (e.g., oxygen, pH) influence its infection site.

2. Explain the difference between **infection** and **inflammation**.

BACTERIA

3. Identify the bacterial cellular morphology and arrangement using the following terms:

bacillus	spirilla	spirochete
staph(ylo)	diplo	strep(to)
pleiomorphic	coccus	tetrad
palisade	Vibrio	

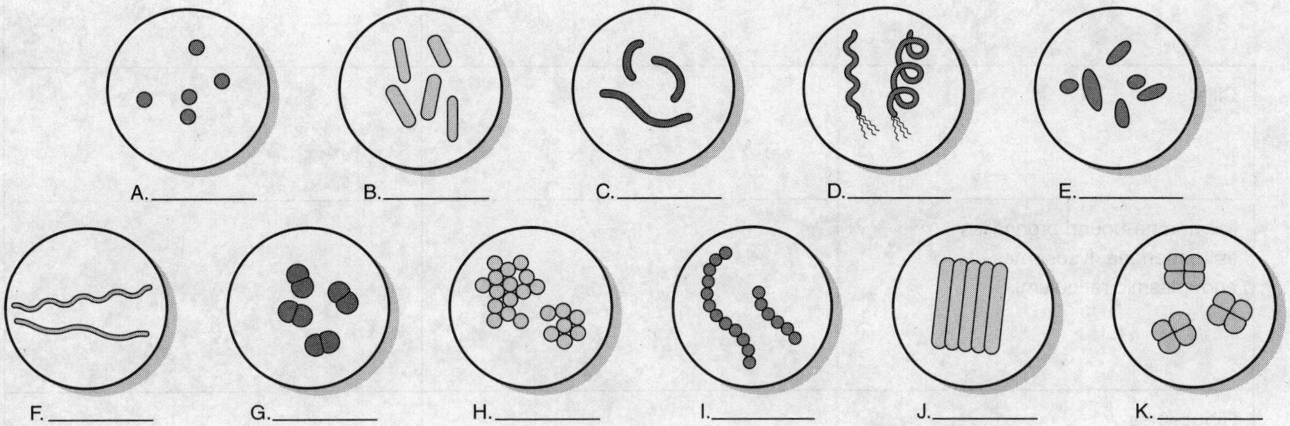

4. Describe the **basic structure** of a bacterium, including cell wall, cell membrane, and its contents.

5. Compare Gram-positive and Gram-negative bacteria based on cell wall structure and staining.

6. Some bacteria secrete toxins. Explain the differences between **exotoxins** and **endotoxins**.

7. What is an **endospore** or **bacterial spore**? Describe the process of spore formation and name genera like *Clostridium* and *Bacillus*.

8. Explain the steps of **binary fission** and its role in bacterial growth.

Copyright © 2027 by Elsevier, Inc. All rights are reserved,
including those for text and data mining, AI training, and similar technologies.

9. Bacterial cells differ from human (eukaryotic) cells in a number of significant ways. Compare and contrast bacterial and eukaryotic cells, using the following chart:

	Bacterial Cells	Human (Eukaryotic) Cells
Cell wall		
Cell membrane		
Capsule or slime coat		
Flagella		
Pili or fimbriae		
Cilia		
Membrane-bound organelles (mitochondria, lysosomes, endoplasmic reticulum)		
Ribosomes		
Nucleus		
Number of chromosomes		
Method of reproduction		

Copyright © 2027 by Elsevier, Inc. All rights are reserved, including those for text and data mining, AI training, and similar technologies.

VIRUSES

10. Why are viruses said to be **"obligate intracellular parasites"**?

11. Describe the **structure** of a viral particle or virion.

12. Outline the basic steps of **viral infection/replication**.

FUNGI

13. Describe the basic structures of the single-cellular and multicellular forms of a fungus.

14. Compare and contrast bacteria, fungi, and viruses using the following chart:

	Bacteria	Fungus	Virus
Basic structure			
Method of reproduction			
Method of culturing			
Drugs used to treat			

OTHER MICROORGANISMS

15. List specific pathological conditions caused by each of the following types of organisms:

   i. chlamydiae:

   ii. rickettsiae:

   iii. mycoplasmas:

   iv. protozoa:

Copyright © 2027 by Elsevier, Inc. All rights are reserved, including those for text and data mining, AI training, and similar technologies.

16. What is a **helminth**? Name an example of a helminth.

17. What is a **prion** and how is it transmitted? Name a human disease caused by a prion.

18. What is meant by the term "normal flora" or "resident flora"?

19. Identify areas of the body that lack resident flora and therefore should be sterile.

20. Explain what is meant by an **endemic infection**.

21. Define a pandemic and name some examples in the last 100 years. Furthermore, describe the COVID-19 pandemic and the unique control measures that have been and are still applied.

22. Define the terms **pathogenicity** and **virulence**. Identify factors that increase the virulence of microorganisms.

CONSOLIDATION OF MICROBIOLOGY

23. Identify the causative agent or agents for each of the following infections. Use the choices listed below.

bacteria	**chlamydia**
fungi	**protozoa**
rickettsiae	**viruses**

i. *Pneumocystis carinii* pneumonia:

ii. candidiasis:

iii. syphilis:

iv. trichomoniasis:

v. tuberculosis:

vi. pneumonia:

vii. tetanus:

viii. Rocky Mountain spotted fever:

ix. tinea pedis:

Copyright © 2027 by Elsevier, Inc. All rights are reserved, including those for text and data mining, AI training, and similar technologies.

x. herpes simplex:

xi. influenza:

xii. botulism:

CONTROL OF TRANSMISSION AND INFECTION

24. What is the basic difference between a disinfectant and an antiseptic?

25. Identify the components in the infection chain and ways in which the cycle can be broken.

26. Describe the methods for determining the effectiveness of an antimicrobial agent as a possible treatment for a specific infection.

27. Define the following terms related to **antibacterial drugs**:

    i. spectrum:

    ii. bacterial resistance:

    iii. bactericidal:

    iv. bacteriostatic:

28. Explain what is meant by the term **superinfection**. What type of microorganism often causes superinfections? Explain how this happens.

29. Describe some of the potential **adverse effects** associated with the use of antibacterial drugs.

30. What is the difference between a **superinfection** and an **opportunistic infection**?

31. When is it appropriate for a physician to prescribe a **narrow spectrum antibacterial** drug?

32. If an antibacterial drug is bacteriostatic rather than bactericidal, how does the individual ever destroy the infecting microorganism?

33. When would the prescription of a bacteriostatic drug not be advisable?

Copyright © 2027 by Elsevier, Inc. All rights are reserved,
including those for text and data mining, AI training, and similar technologies.

34. Explain how the **misuse or overuse** of antibacterial agents could lead to the development of bacterial resistance.

35. If antibacterial drugs are not effective in the treatment of viral infections, why are they often prescribed for individuals with chronic viral infections such as hepatitis B, hepatitis C, or HIV?

36. Identify guidelines that an individual should follow to **maximize the effects** of antibacterial medications.

37. Explain why it has been difficult to develop **antiviral drugs**.

38. How do **interferons** contribute to preventing viral spread, and what is their potential role in treatment?

39. Explain the physiological impact of a systemic bacterial infection like **septicemia** on the body.

Copyright © 2027 by Elsevier, Inc. All rights are reserved,
including those for text and data mining, AI training, and similar technologies.

7 Immunity

1. State the three main components of the immune system and identify the cells/tissues/organs in each of the components.

2. Match the terms with the structures/organs.

Bone marrow	Lymphatic vessels
Lymph nodes – axillary	Palatine tonsil
Lymph nodes – cervical	Pharyngeal tonsil (adenoid)
Lymph nodes – inguinal	Spleen
Lymph nodes – intestinal	Thymus

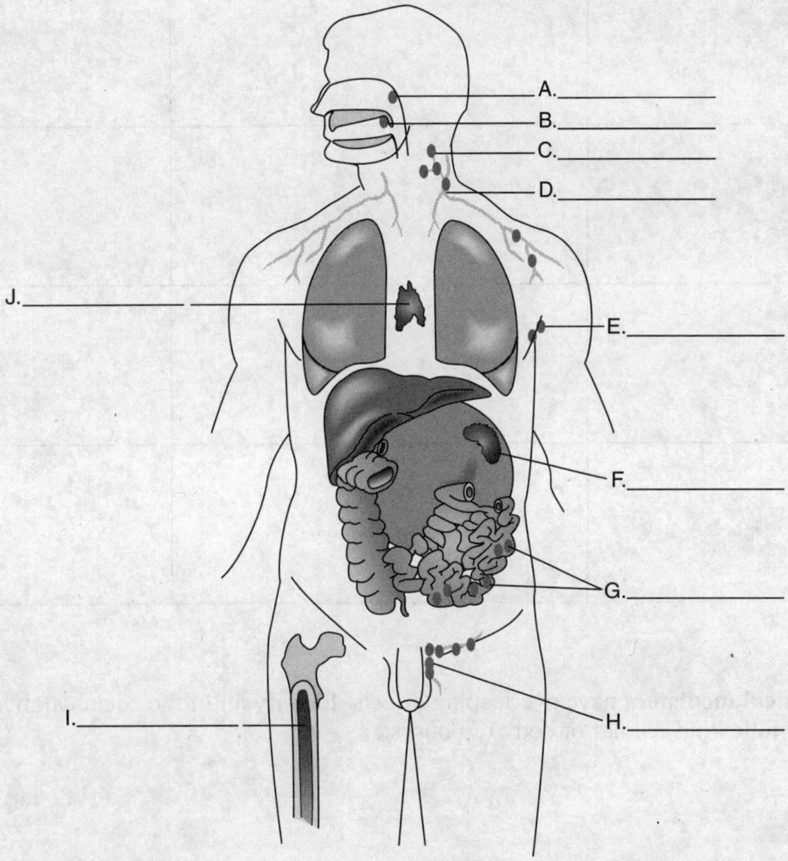

Copyright © 2027 by Elsevier, Inc. All rights are reserved, including those for text and data mining, AI training, and similar technologies.

3. What is a **cell surface antigen**? Why is it important?

4. What is the major histocompatibility complex, and how is it related to the human leukocyte antigens?

5. Chemical mediators play an important role in both inflammation and immunity. Identify the source and effects of the major chemical mediators using the following chart:

Chemical Mediator	Source	Effects
Histamine		
Prostaglandins		
Cytokines (lymphokines, monokines, interleukins, interferon)		
Leukotrienes		
Kinins (bradykinin)		
Complement		

6. Several of the **chemical mediators** have overlapping effects. Identify all of the chemical mediators that are responsible for each of the following cellular or body responses:

   i. vasodilation:

   ii. increased capillary permeability:

Copyright © 2027 by Elsevier, Inc. All rights are reserved, including those for text and data mining, AI training, and similar technologies.

iii. chemotaxis:

iv. pain:

v. contraction of bronchiolar walls/bronchospasm:

vi. proliferation of leukocytes:

vii. pruritus:

viii. fever:

7. All of the following cells are involved in immunity. Identify the role of each.

Cell Type	Function
Macrophages	
Natural killer cells	
T lymphocytes	
Cytotoxic or killer T cells	
Helper T cells (T4 or CD4 lymphocytes)	
Memory T cells	
Suppressor T cells (T8)	
B lymphocytes	
Plasma cells	
B memory cells	

8. Which cells participate in **both** cellular and humoral immunity?

Copyright © 2027 by Elsevier, Inc. All rights are reserved,
including those for text and data mining, AI training, and similar technologies.

9. Match the five **classes of antibodies or immunoglobulins with their chemical structure** and state the functions of each.

IgA

IgD

IgE

IgG

IgM

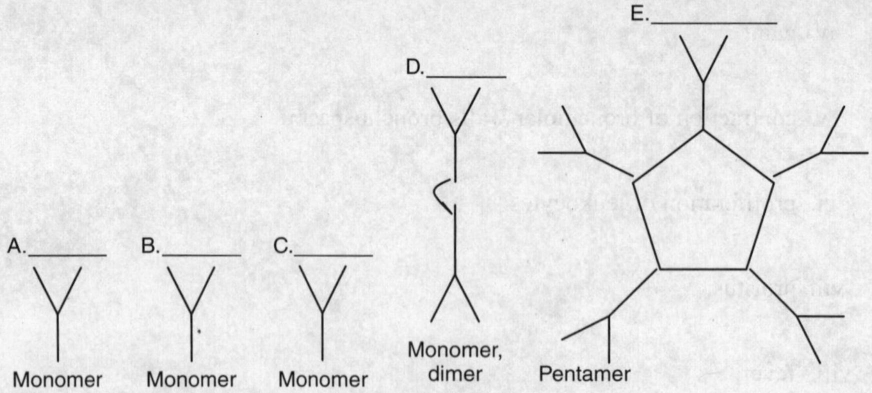

10. Explain how antibodies exert their effects and how the release of complement contributes to these effects.

11. What is the approximate time frame between exposure to an antigen and the appearance of immunoglobulins in the serum on the first exposure to a specific antigen? On subsequent exposure to the antigen?

12. What is the average length of time required to acquire an **effective antibody titer** following exposure to an antigen on first exposure and subsequent exposures?

13. Explain the action of an mRNA vaccine.

14. What is a cytokine storm and what can trigger such an event?

15. Explain the rationale for "boosters."

16. Explain why individuals may contract infections such as colds, influenza, and sexually transmitted diseases repeatedly.

Copyright © 2027 by Elsevier, Inc. All rights are reserved, including those for text and data mining, AI training, and similar technologies.

17. Compare and contrast active and passive immunity using the following chart:

Characteristic	Active Immunity	Passive Immunity
Method of acquisition		
Onset of immunity after exposure to antigen		
Duration of effectiveness		
Examples		

18. A serious complication of organ transplantation is **organ rejection**. Identify measures that are taken in an attempt to prevent this from happening.

19. A common adverse effect of immunosuppressant drugs is the development of "**opportunistic infections**." What is meant by the term "opportunistic"? Explain how this complication occurs.

20. What medications are often prescribed prophylactically for an individual who is taking immunosuppressant drugs? Explain the rationale.

Copyright © 2027 by Elsevier, Inc. All rights are reserved, including those for text and data mining, AI training, and similar technologies.

HYPERSENSITIVITY

21. Compare and contrast the different **types of hypersensitivity** reactions using the following chart:

Type	Mechanism	Effects	Example
I			
II			
III			
IV			

22. Hypovolemic shock is a potential complication of extensive burns (see Chapter 12). Compare and contrast this type of shock with anaphylactic shock using the following chart:

	Hypovolemic Shock	Anaphylactic Shock
Etiology		
Distinguishing features		
Specific treatment		

Copyright © 2027 by Elsevier, Inc. All rights are reserved, including those for text and data mining, AI training, and similar technologies.

23. List the types of medications that might be prescribed in the **treatment of allergic conditions**.

24. Identify and describe the type of reaction(s) involved in latex hypersensitivity.

AUTOIMMUNITY

25. State the underlying mechanism responsible for **autoimmune disorders**.

26. How is **systemic lupus erythematosus** diagnosed?

27. What types of **medications and therapeutic interventions** might be prescribed in the treatment of the autoimmune disorder systemic lupus erythematosus? Explain the rationale for each treatment.

28. Systemic lupus erythematosus has widespread effects virtually throughout the body. Identify common manifestations under the following headings:

    i. skin:

    ii. joints:

    iii. heart:

    iv. blood vessels:

    v. blood/bone marrow:

    vi. kidneys:

    vii. lungs:

    viii. central nervous system:

IMMUNODEFICIENCY

29. List common causes of **immunodeficiency**.

Copyright © 2027 by Elsevier, Inc. All rights are reserved,
including those for text and data mining, AI training, and similar technologies.

30. Identify the **general effects of immunodeficiency**.

31. Identify the types of **medications** that are often prescribed for the immunodeficient individual or immunocompromised host and explain the rationale for each drug group.

HIV AND AIDS

32. What is the **causative agent** responsible for **AIDS**? Describe its properties.

33. Which cells are targeted by HIV? Identify the consequences of this.

34. List the **routes of transmission** of HIV.

35. Identify individuals who are at **high risk** for contracting HIV.

36. What is the average "window" or **incubation period** for HIV? State the possible **range**.

37. How is a **diagnosis of HIV infection** confirmed?

38. What is the average length of time between infection with HIV and development of **full-blown AIDS**?

39. How is a **diagnosis of AIDS** confirmed?

40. Identify possible manifestations of the **initial phase of HIV** infection.

41. As HIV progresses and the individual's immune system becomes more compromised, literally every bodily system is affected. Describe these complications under the following headings:

    i. generalized effects:

    ii. opportunistic infections:

    iii. gastrointestinal manifestations:

    iv. oral manifestations:

Copyright © 2027 by Elsevier, Inc. All rights are reserved, including those for text and data mining, AI training, and similar technologies.

v. respiratory manifestations:

vi. nervous system manifestations:

vii. malignancies:

42. Identify **medications** that are used in the treatment of an individual with HIV and AIDS, including those that are prescribed to prevent potential complications.

43. What is the **prognosis** for an individual infected with HIV?

Copyright © 2027 by Elsevier, Inc. All rights are reserved,
including those for text and data mining, AI training, and similar technologies.

8 Skin Disorders

1. Identify the five primary functions of skin and explain how each contributes to overall body homeostasis.

2. Match structures of the skin with the terms provided.

Adipose tissue, Artery, Capillaries, Dermis, Eccrine gland, Epidermis, Hair, Hair follicle, Melanocyte, Nerve fiber, Sebaceous gland, Sensory receptor, Smooth muscle, Stratum basale, Stratum corneum, Subcutaneous tissue, Vein

A. ____________________

B. ____________________

C. ____________________

D. ____________________

E. ____________________

F. ____________________

G. ____________________

H. ____________________

I. ____________________

J. ____________________

K. ____________________

L. ____________________

M. ____________________

N. ____________________

O. ____________________

P. ____________________

Q. ____________________

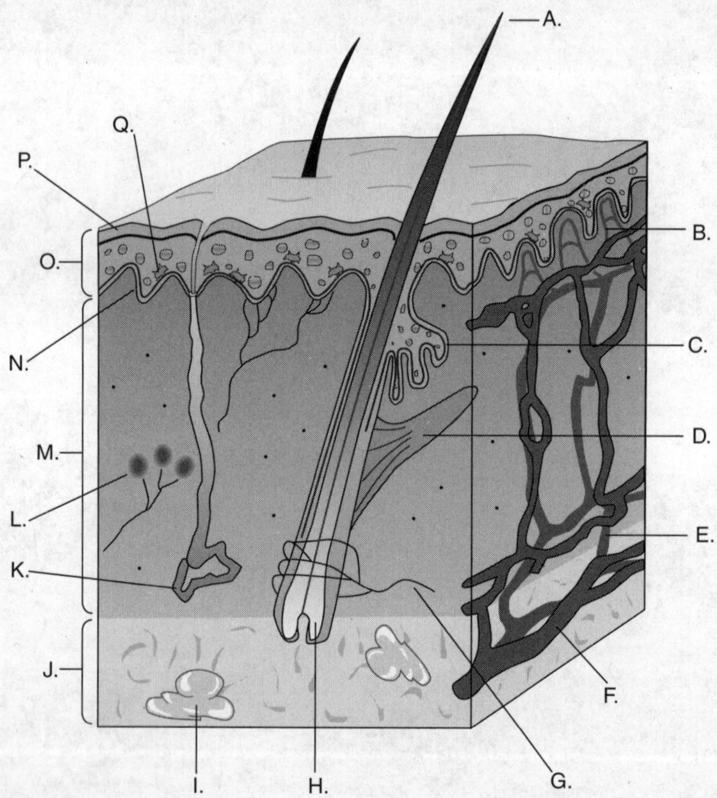

Copyright © 2027 by Elsevier, Inc. All rights are reserved, including those for text and data mining, AI training, and similar technologies.

3. Explain the role of melanocytes in skin protection.

4. Describe how sebaceous and eccrine glands aid skin function.

5. State the **etiology** and **treatment** for each of the following skin conditions. Be as specific as possible. If the cause is an infection, identify the causative organism.

Condition	Etiology	Treatment
Scleroderma		
Kaposi sarcoma		
Tinea		
Atopic dermatitis		
Pemphigus		
Herpes simplex		
Verruca		
Urticaria		
Psoriasis		
Scabies		
Impetigo		
Cellulitis		
Necrotizing fasciitis		

Copyright © 2027 by Elsevier, Inc. All rights reserved,
including those for text and data mining, AI training, and similar technologies.

6. Identify individuals who are at **high risk** for developing each of the following **malignancies**:

   i. squamous cell carcinoma:

   ii. malignant melanoma:

   iii. Kaposi sarcoma:

7. List the four warning signs of skin cancer.

8. Describe diagnostic tests for skin lesions, including biopsy.

9. Match common skin lesions with the terms provided.

   (Fissure, Macule, Nodule, Papule, Plaque, Pustule, Ulcer, Vesicle)

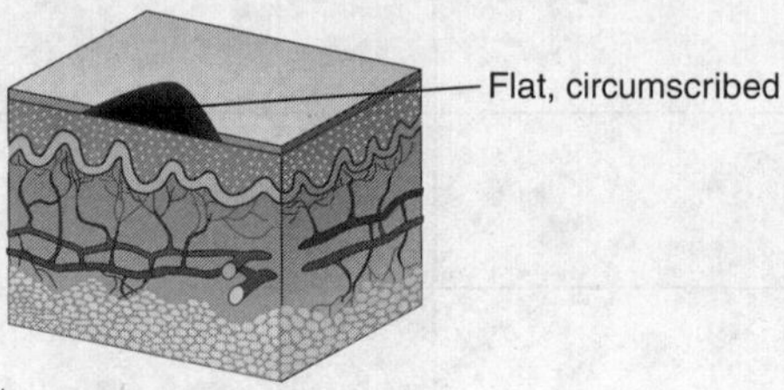

A. ____________

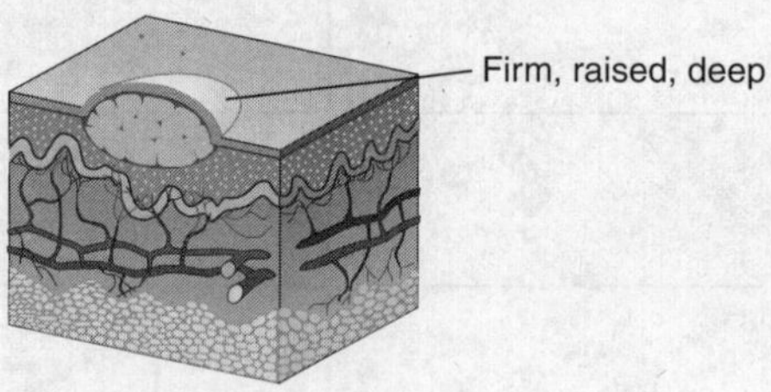

B. ____________

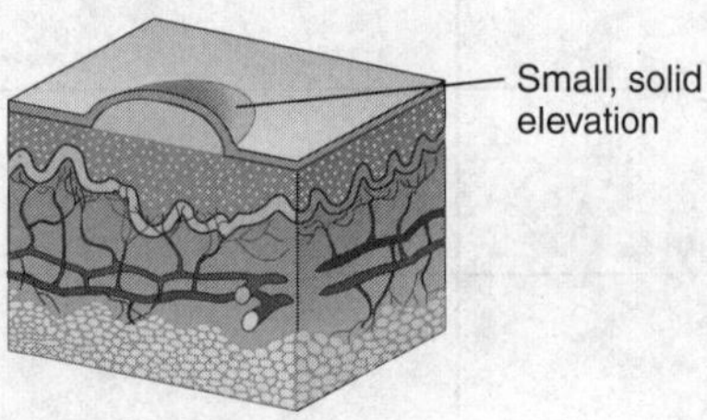

C. ____________

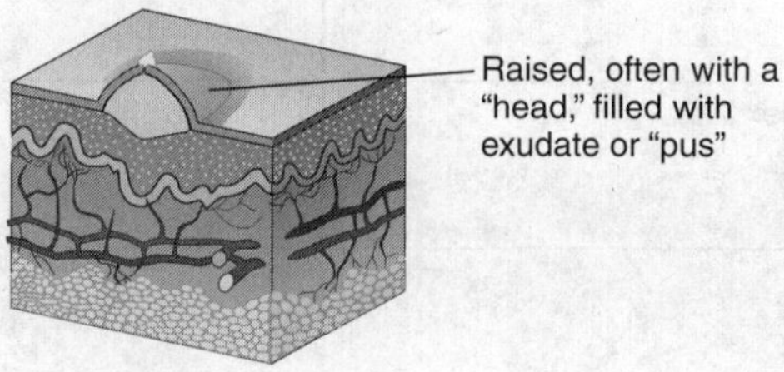

D. ____________

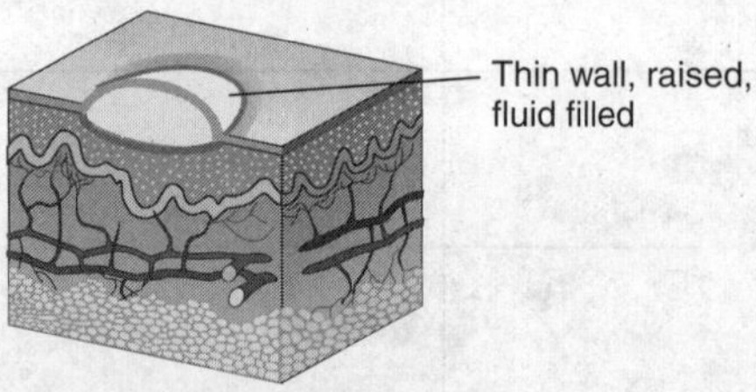

E. ____________

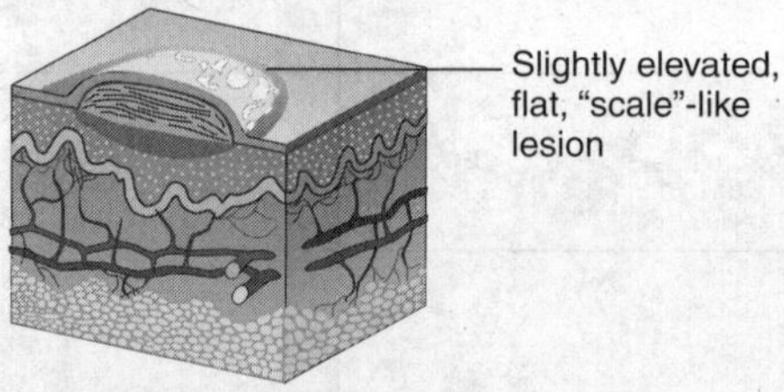

F. ____________

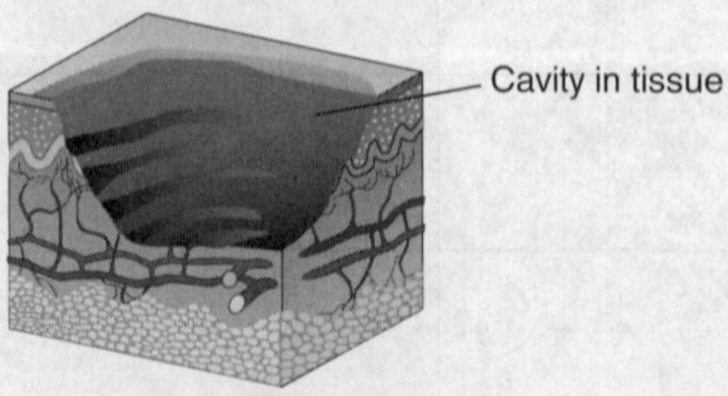

G. ____________

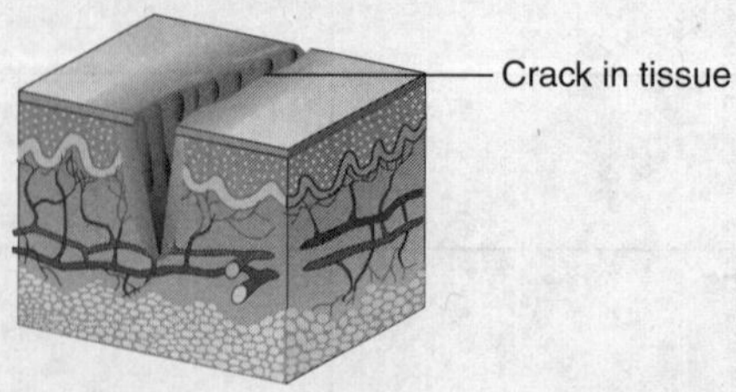

H. ____________

Copyright © 2027 by Elsevier, Inc. All rights reserved, including those for text and data mining, AI training, and similar technologies.

CONSOLIDATION

10. Identify the disease or diseases for which each of the following statements or characteristics is true:

    i. most commonly associated with HIV and AIDS:

    ii. commonly known as hives:

    iii. an autoimmune disorder that results in blister formation:

    iv. caused by a mite:

    v. commonly known as cold sores:

    vi. caused by human papillomavirus:

    vii. superficial fungal infection:

    viii. commonly known as eczema:

    ix. hand deformity involving excess tissue growth under the skin of palm:

11. List three skin cancer prevention measures.

Copyright © 2027 by Elsevier, Inc. All rights are reserved,
including those for text and data mining, AI training, and similar technologies.

9 Musculoskeletal System Disorders

FRACTURES

1. Match the parts of a long bone with the following terms.

Articular cartilage, Compact bone, Diaphysis, Endosteum, Epiphyseal line, Epiphysis, Medullary cavity, Nutrient foramen, Periosteum, Spongy bone

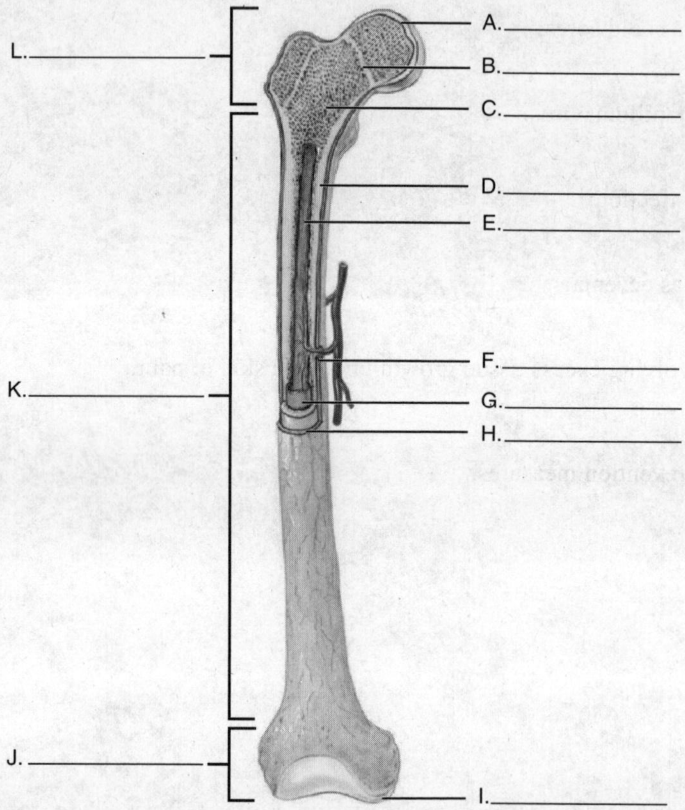

From Applegate EJ: *The anatomy and physiology learning system,* ed 4, St. Louis, 2011, Saunders.

Copyright © 2027 by Elsevier, Inc. All rights are reserved, including those for text and data mining, AI training, and similar technologies.

2. Outline the **distinguishing characteristics** of the following types of fractures and match the type of fracture with the diagrams.

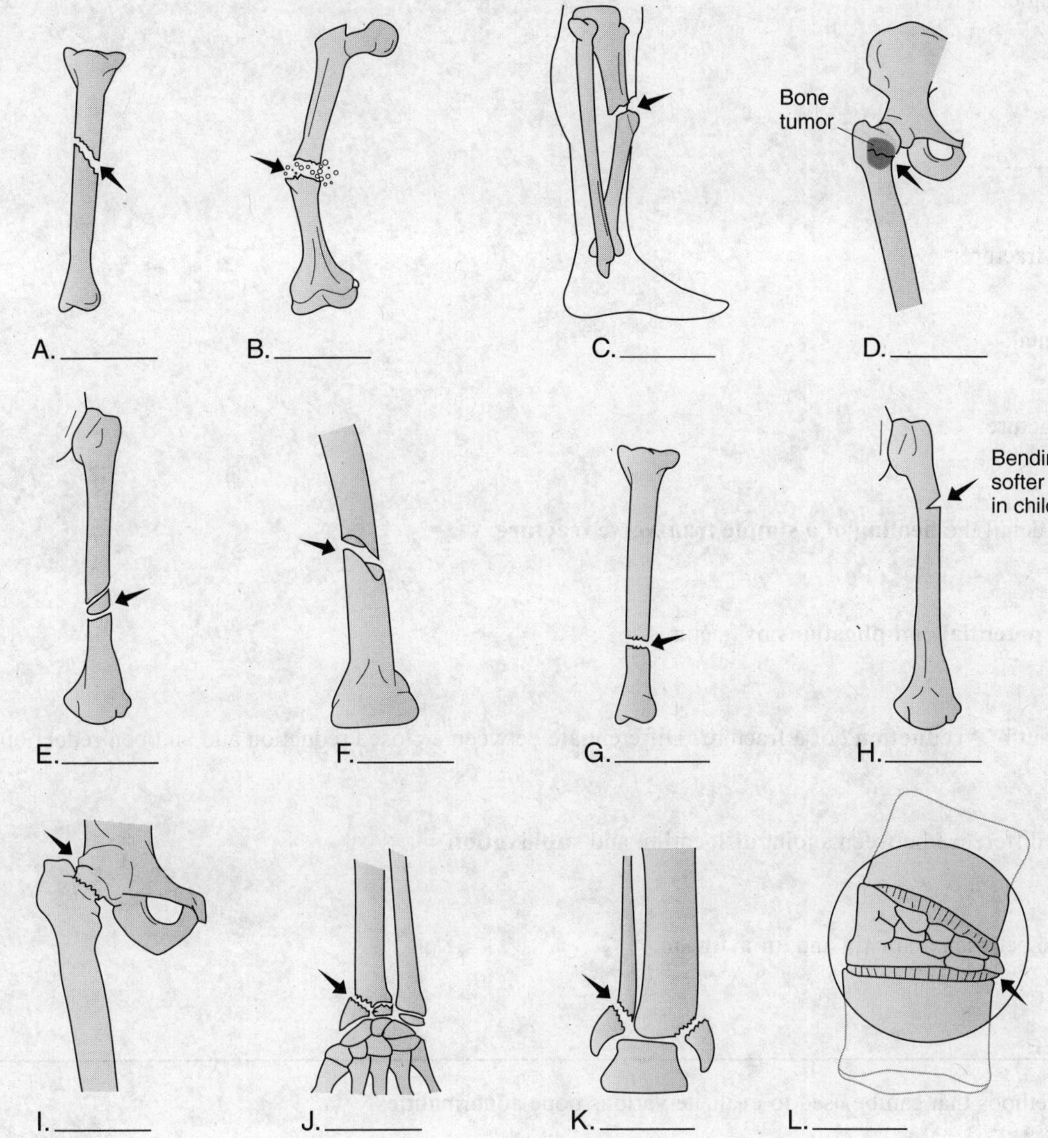

i. open:

ii. comminuted:

iii. compression:

iv. greenstick:

v. impacted:

Copyright © 2027 by Elsevier, Inc. All rights are reserved, including those for text and data mining, AI training, and similar technologies.

vi. oblique:

vii. pathological:

viii. spiral:

ix. transverse:

x. Colles fracture:

xi. segmental:

xii. Pott fracture:

3. Describe in detail the **healing of a simple transverse fracture**.

4. Identify the **potential complications** of fractures.

5. What is meant by **"reduction"** of a fracture? Differentiate between a closed reduction and an open reduction.

6. Explain the difference between a joint **dislocation** and **subluxation**.

7. Differentiate between **a sprain** and **an avulsion**.

BONE DISEASE

8. Identify methods that can be used to evaluate various bone abnormalities.

9. List factors that **predispose** an individual to osteoporosis.

10. Identify **common sites** of osteoporosis.

11. Identify the condition **osteopenia** as it relates to osteoporosis.

12. Describe the **pathophysiology** of osteoporosis.

Copyright © 2027 by Elsevier, Inc. All rights are reserved, including those for text and data mining, AI training, and similar technologies.

13. Outline the **treatment** of osteoporosis, including the rationale for each therapeutic intervention.

14. Complete the following chart comparing and contrasting **rickets, osteomalacia,** and **Paget disease**:

	Rickets	Osteomalacia	Paget Disease
Etiology			
Manifestations			
Treatment			

15. Identify a drug group that may cause osteomalacia with prolonged use.

16. Differentiate between **an osteosarcoma** and **a chondrosarcoma**.

MUSCULAR DYSTROPHY

17. Describe the basic **pathology** involved in muscular dystrophy.

18. Complete the following chart comparing and contrasting the four types of **muscular dystrophy**:

	Duchenne	Fascioscapulo-Humeral	Myotonic	Limb Girdle
Mode of inheritance				
Age of onset				
Muscle involvement				
Progression				

Copyright © 2027 by Elsevier, Inc. All rights are reserved,
including those for text and data mining, AI training, and similar technologies.

PRIMARY FIBROMYALGIA SYNDROME

19. Identify the **manifestations** of fibromyalgia.

ARTHRITIS

20. Explain why osteoarthritis is often referred to as **"wear-and-tear" arthritis.**

21. How is osteoarthritis diagnosed?

22. Complete the following chart comparing osteoarthritis and rheumatoid arthritis:

	Osteoarthritis	Rheumatoid Arthritis
Etiology		
Predisposing factors		
Joints involved		
Pathophysiology		
Signs and symptoms		
Systemic effects		
Treatment		

23. Identify **drug types** that may be used in the treatment of rheumatoid arthritis.

24. Outline how **juvenile rheumatoid arthritis** differs from the adult form.

25. Identify unique manifestation associated with **psoriatic arthritis**.

26. Identify the basic underlying problem with **gout**.

27. Outline how gout differs from other forms of arthritis.

28. Describe the **pathological changes** that occur in **ankylosing spondylitis**.

Copyright © 2027 by Elsevier, Inc. All rights reserved, including those for text and data mining, AI training, and similar technologies.

CONSOLIDATION

29. Identify the disease or diseases for which each of the following statements or characteristics is true:

i. loss of articular cartilage:

ii. development of tophi in soft tissue, bone, or both:

iii. possible presence of an antibody against IgG in the serum:

iv. classified as an autoimmune disease:

v. presence of extraarticular (i.e., systemic) manifestations:

vi. a sex-linked disorder:

vii. may be treated with bisphosphonates:

viii. most commonly affects weight-bearing joints:

ix. highest incidence in women between the ages of 20 and 50:

x. characterized by synovitis and pannus formation:

xi. treatment may involve intraarticular injections of glucocorticoids:

xii. may result in the development of kyphosis:

xiii. may be accompanied by ocular complications such as uveitis:

xiv. affects joints in hands and feet:

xv. characterized by elevated serum uric acid levels:

xvi. development of ankylosis or joint fusion over time:

xvii. treated with NSAIDs:

xviii. immunosuppressants sometimes prescribed during exacerbations:

xix. characterized by the development of osteophytes:

Copyright © 2027 by Elsevier, Inc. All rights are reserved,
including those for text and data mining, AI training, and similar technologies.

xx. primary involvement occurs in the intervertebral joints:

xxi. characterized by compression fractures of the vertebral bodies:

xxii. crepitus often present:

xxiii. treated with additional vitamin D and calcium:

xxiv. general term referring to severe inflammation and subsequent damage of the muscles:

Copyright © 2027 by Elsevier, Inc. All rights are reserved, including those for text and data mining, AI training, and similar technologies.

10 Blood and Circulatory System Disorders

ERYTHROCYTES

1. Describe the normal **"life cycle"** of an erythrocyte, including its site of production, average life span, and the process of its destruction and breakdown.

2. State the normal range for both **red blood cell count** and **hemoglobin**, differentiating between the values found in males and females.

3. Define **anemia**.

4. List the general manifestations that result from all types of anemias.

5. Complete the following chart comparing the different types of anemias:

Type of Anemia	Etiology	Specific Signs and Symptoms	Specific Treatment
Iron deficiency anemia			
Pernicious anemia—vitamin B_{12} deficiency anemia			
Aplastic anemia			
Thalassemia			
Sickle cell anemia			

6. **Sickle cell anemia** is an inherited disorder. What is the pattern of inheritance for this disorder, and what is the genotype of an individual with sickle cell anemia?

Copyright © 2027 by Elsevier, Inc. All rights are reserved, including those for text and data mining, AI training, and similar technologies.

7. What is meant by the **"sickle cell trait"**? What is the genotype of an individual who has this trait?

8. A woman with sickle cell trait is pregnant with the child of a man who has sickle cell anemia. Draw a Punnett square to illustrate possible outcomes:

   i. What is the probability that the child will have sickle cell anemia?

   ii. What is the probability that the child will have sickle cell trait?

   iii. What is the probability that the child will have neither sickle cell trait nor sickle cell anemia?

   iv. What is the probability that any future child that this couple conceives will have sickle cell anemia?

9. Describe the **pathophysiology** of sickle cell anemia.

10. What precipitates **"sickling"**?

11. What is meant by a **"crisis"**? Identify the potential complications of a sickling crisis.

12. Explain why an individual with sickle cell anemia may experience the following signs and symptoms:

    i. jaundice:

    ii. cerebrovascular accident:

    iii. frequent infections:

    iv. splenomegaly:

    v. congestive heart failure:

13. Is there any means of preventing sickle cell anemia?

14. Define **polycythemia**.

15. Differentiate between **primary** and **secondary polycythemia**.

Copyright © 2027 by Elsevier, Inc. All rights are reserved, including those for text and data mining, AI training, and similar technologies.

16. Describe the signs, symptoms, and **complications of polycythemia**.

17. Identify three therapeutic interventions used in the **treatment of polycythemia**.

BLOOD CLOTTING

18. Draw a flow chart representing the three steps involved in **blood coagulation**.

19. List the warning signs of excessive bleeding and possible clotting disorders.

20. Describe diagnostic tests that can be employed to identify and/or monitor bleeding disorders.

21. Identify six causes of abnormal bleeding, explaining how each interferes with normal hemostasis.

22. Explain how and why each of the following factors would affect **hemostasis** (i.e., promote or delay blood clotting):

    i. liver disease:

    ii. ingestion of aspirin:

    iii. prolonged antibiotic therapy:

    iv. administration of heparin:

    v. vitamin K deficiency:

    vi. prolonged inactivity (e.g., postoperatively or sitting on a plane for many hours):

    vii. polycythemia:

    viii. thrombocytopenia:

    ix. increased hematocrit:

    x. administration of warfarin (Coumadin):

23. **Hemophilia A** is an inherited disorder. What is the specific clotting factor deficit, and what is the pattern of inheritance?

Copyright © 2027 by Elsevier, Inc. All rights are reserved, including those for text and data mining, AI training, and similar technologies.

24. A woman is a carrier for hemophilia A. She is pregnant with the child of a man who does not have hemophilia. What is her genotype for this disorder? Draw a Punnett square to show possible outcomes.

i. What is the probability that the child she is carrying will have hemophilia A? Would a child with hemophilia be a male or female?

ii. What is the probability that the child will be a carrier of hemophilia? What would be the sex of a child who is a carrier?

iii. What is the probability that the child will neither have hemophilia nor be a carrier of the disease?

iv. What is the probability that any future sons whom this couple conceives will have hemophilia?

v. What is the probability that any future daughters whom this couple conceives will be carriers of hemophilia?

25. A man with hemophilia A marries a woman whose father has hemophilia A.

i. What is the man's genotype?

ii. What is his wife's genotype?

Draw a Punnett square to illustrate the genotypes of possible children.

i. What is the probability that any children whom this couple produces will have hemophilia?

ii. What is the probability that any children whom this couple produces will be carriers of hemophilia?

iii. What will be the sex of a child who is a carrier?

26. Describe the pathophysiology of **Disseminated Intravascular Coagulation**, explaining how it involves both excessive clotting and bleeding.

LEUKOCYTES

27. Define **leukemia**.

28. What is a "blast" cell? Describe its characteristics.

29. Explain the two **major classifications** of leukemia.

Copyright © 2027 by Elsevier, Inc. All rights are reserved, including those for text and data mining, AI training, and similar technologies.

30. Identify individuals who are considered at high risk for the development of leukemia.

31. What test could be used to confirm a diagnosis of leukemia?

32. The signs and symptoms of leukemia are diverse and widespread throughout the body. Explain why each of the signs and symptoms occurs:

i. weight loss and fatigue:

ii. anemia:

iii. thrombocytopenia:

iv. multiple infections, including those caused by microorganisms of low virulence:

v. increased bleeding and even severe hemorrhage:

vi. kidney stones:

vii. fever:

viii. lymphadenopathy:

ix. splenomegaly and hepatomegaly:

x. bone pain:

33. Describe the treatments used for the client with leukemia, including the adverse effects or complications of each.

34. Describe the different **prognoses** for the types of leukemia.

Copyright © 2027 by Elsevier, Inc. All rights are reserved, including those for text and data mining, AI training, and similar technologies.

35. Complete the following chart comparing acute and chronic leukemia:

	Acute Leukemia	Chronic Leukemia
Age of onset		
Course of disease		
Severity of symptoms		
Number of blast cells		
Response to treatment		

ATHEROSCLEROSIS

36. Describe four general treatment measures for cardiac disorders.

37. Identify nine risk factors for developing atherosclerosis. Indicate which ones are modifiable and which ones are not. Note that these are the same risk factors for heart disease.

38. Describe the process of **atheroma formation** in atherosclerosis, from endothelial injury to the formation of a complicated plaque.

39. Describe the significance of plaque formation, including five potential **complications of atherosclerosis**.

40. Which vessels are affected by atherosclerosis?

41. Describe common therapeutic interventions, to include lifestyle changes, used in the treatment of atherosclerosis.

42. Explain the rationale for prescribing the following drugs:

i. antilipidemics or lipid-lowering drugs:

ii. platelet inhibitors:

iii. anticoagulants:

iv. antihypertensives:

Copyright © 2027 by Elsevier, Inc. All rights are reserved, including those for text and data mining, AI training, and similar technologies.

43. What type of surgical interventions can be used in advanced atheromas?

44. What are the key signs and symptoms of peripheral vascular disease in the legs?

45. Describe the pathophysiology of varicose veins, including the role of weak vein walls and damaged valves.

46. Differentiate between thrombophlebitis and phlebothrombosis. What critical problem can arise from venous thrombosis?

CONSOLIDATION

47. For each of the following characteristics, identify the blood disorder or disorders in which they occur:

i. involves both excessive bleeding and clotting:

ii. decreased or lack of intrinsic factor production:

iii. characterized by primitive blast cells:

iv. sex-linked bleeding disorder:

v. increased production of erythrocytes:

vi. frequent adverse effect of chemotherapy:

vii. may result in impaired growth and development:

viii. common in individuals from the Mediterranean area:

ix. may be accompanied by jaundice:

x. may be accompanied by loss of coordination:

xi. a neoplastic disorder involving the red blood cells:

xii. more prevalent in individuals with Down syndrome:

xiii. predisposes individuals to infections:

Copyright © 2027 by Elsevier, Inc. All rights are reserved,
including those for text and data mining, AI training, and similar technologies.

11 Lymphatic System Disorders

LYMPHATIC SYSTEM STRUCTURES

1. Match the terms with the structures/organs of the lymphatic system in the figure.

   Arteriole, Axillary lymph nodes, Blood capillary, Bone marrow, Inguinal lymph nodes, Left subclavian vein, Lymph capillaries, Right lymphatic duct, Right subclavian vein, Spleen, Thoracic duct, Thymus, Tissue cells, Tonsil, Venule

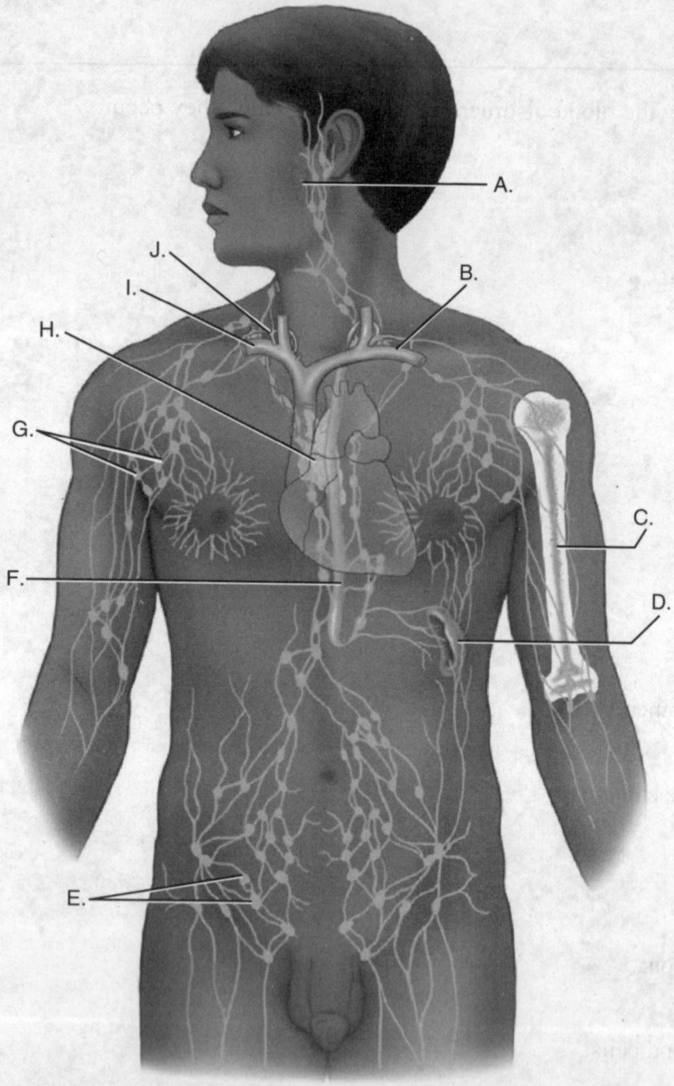

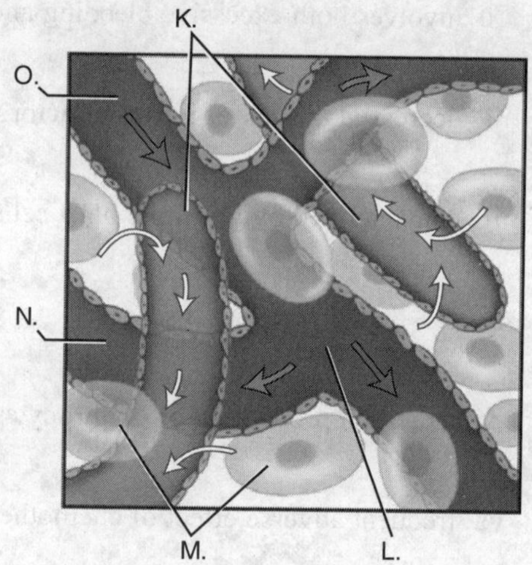

From VanMeter K, Hubert R: *Microbiology for the healthcare professional,* ed 3, St. Louis, 2022, Elsevier.

Copyright © 2027 by Elsevier, Inc. All rights reserved, including those for text and data mining, AI training, and similar technologies.

A. ____________________ I. ____________________

B. ____________________ J. ____________________

C. ____________________ K. ____________________

D. ____________________ L. ____________________

E. ____________________ M. ____________________

F. ____________________ N. ____________________

G. ____________________ O. ____________________

H. ____________________

LYMPHATIC SYSTEM DISORDERS

2. What type of cell forms the diagnosis for Hodgkin disease? Describe this cell.

3. Outline the basis for the staging of Hodgkin disease.

4. Describe the signs and symptoms of Hodgkin disease through the four stages.

5. Identify treatments for Hodgkin disease.

6. Explain how non-Hodgkin lymphoma differs from Hodgkin disease.

7. Define multiple myeloma.

8. Describe the signs and symptoms of multiple myeloma, including the reason that each occurs.

9. List treatment methods for multiple myeloma.

Copyright © 2027 by Elsevier, Inc. All rights are reserved,
including those for text and data mining, AI training, and similar technologies.

12 Cardiovascular System Disorders

HEART

1. Identify the structures of the heart using the following labels:

aorta
aortic semilunar valve
chordae tendineae
inferior vena cava
interventricular septum
left atrium
left ventricle
mitral (bicuspid valve)
papillary muscle
pericardium
right atrium
right ventricle
superior vena cava

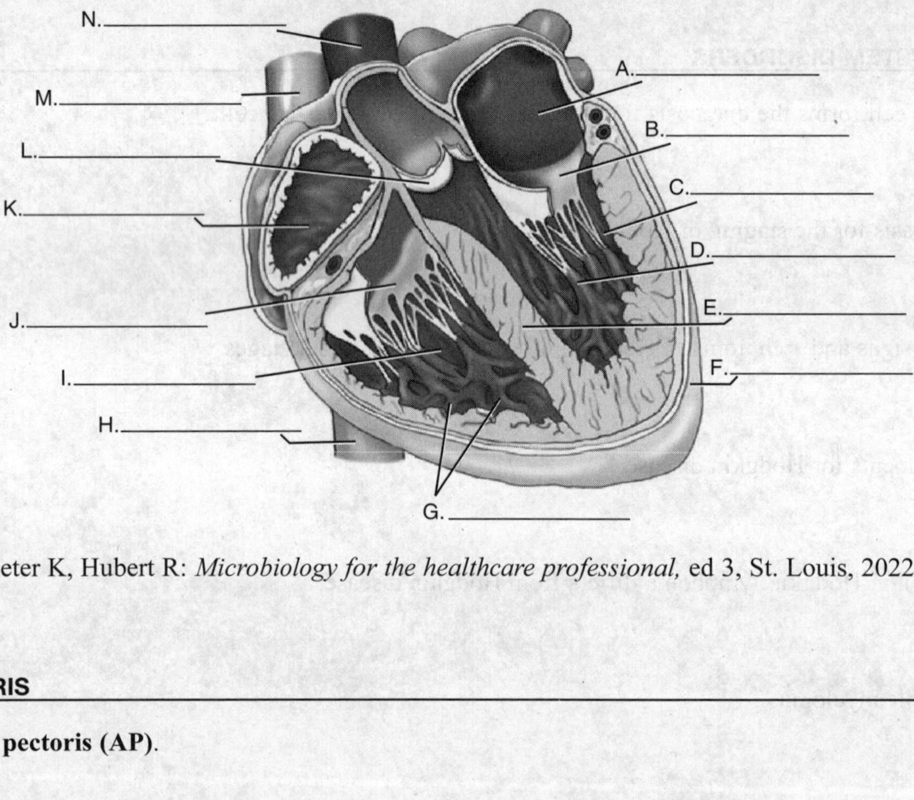

From VanMeter K, Hubert R: *Microbiology for the healthcare professional,* ed 3, St. Louis, 2022, Elsevier.

ANGINA PECTORIS

2. Define **angina pectoris (AP)**.

3. What is the **underlying pathology** involved in AP?

4. Identify three disorders that may **cause** or **predispose** an individual to angina.

Copyright © 2027 by Elsevier, Inc. All rights are reserved, including those for text and data mining, AI training, and similar technologies.

5. What is the **most serious complication** of AP?

6. The factors listed below often **precipitate an attack** (i.e., pain) in an individual with a history of angina. Explain the mechanism involved for each of them:

    i. smoking a cigarette or being exposed to second-hand smoke:

    ii. going from a warm environment into the cold:

    iii. engaging in an argument or other stressful behavior:

    iv. exercise, such as climbing a flight of stairs or running:

7. Describe the classic manifestations of an anginal attack. What is the usual duration of an anginal attack?

8. Identify the primary **drug** used to treat an **acute anginal attack**? Explain how these drugs relieve chest pain.

9. In an emergency angina attack, how would you administer nitroglycerin?

10. Outline the **management of an anginal attack**, including both immediate and preventative measures.

11. When should emergency medical services (EMS) be requested during an anginal attack?

12. The drug groups identified in the accompanying chart are often prescribed alone or in combination to control angina and prevent periods of myocardial hypoxia. Explain the action of each type and how each would prevent anginal pain. Also identify adverse effects and one example for each group.

Drug Group	Action and Effects	Adverse Effects	Example
β-Adrenergic blockers			
Calcium channel blockers			
Nitrates (vasodilators; transdermal or oral form)			

Copyright © 2027 by Elsevier, Inc. All rights are reserved,
including those for text and data mining, AI training, and similar technologies.

13. List **other types of medication** that might be prescribed for an individual with angina and explain the rationale for each.

14. Identify **surgical interventions** that might be used in the treatment of angina.

15. Describe three **nonpharmacological interventions** that could help to control angina.

16. What additional information should be obtained from a patient reporting AP to fully assess their condition?

17. Identify measures that would help decrease the chance of an individual experiencing an **anginal attack**.

MYOCARDIAL INFARCTION

18. Define **myocardial infarction (MI)**.

19. Describe the five types of **MIs**, including their distinguishing characteristics.

20. State three **causes of MI** and indicate which one occurs most frequently.

21. List the **warning signs** of an MI.

22. Differentiate between a transmural and intramural infarction.

23. What is the **most common site** of an MI, and why is this area particularly vulnerable?

24. Describe the **pathophysiology** of an MI, including the role of ischemia and necrosis.

25. Describe the manifestations of an MI.

26. How could a **diagnosis** of MI be **confirmed**?

27. What are **serum enzymes**? What is their significance in someone who has suffered an MI? Differentiate between enzymes and isoenzymes.

28. Explain why the **electrocardiogram (ECG)** would change after an MI.

Copyright © 2027 by Elsevier, Inc. All rights reserved, including those for text and data mining, AI training, and similar technologies.

29. Identify the most common complication of myocardial infarction responsible for the highest mortality rate and explain its severity.

30. Briefly describe **other complications** that may accompany an MI.

31. Identify the treatments for an MI and include the rationale for each.

32. Identify at least four differences between AP and MI regarding etiology, symptoms, and treatment.

CARDIAC DYSRHYTHMIAS (ARRHYTHMIAS)

33. Locate and label the components of the cardiac conduction system on the following diagram:

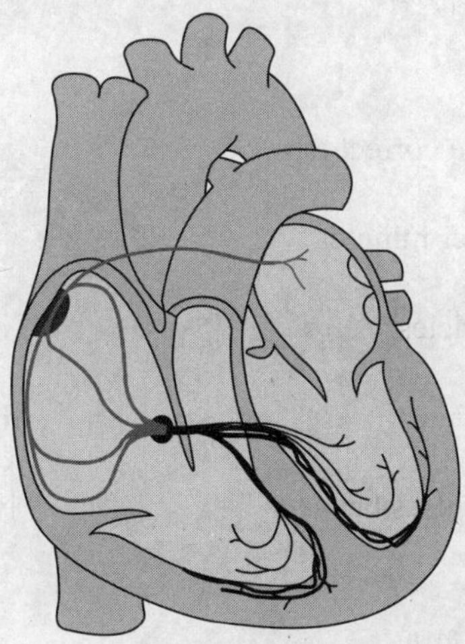

Structures

atrioventricular (AV) bundle (Bundle of His)
AV node
left bundle branch
Purkinje fibers
right bundle branch
sinoatrial (SA) node

34. Describe the pathway of electrical impulses in the cardiac conduction system, starting from the sinoatrial (SA) node.

35. Label the following diagram of an ECG:

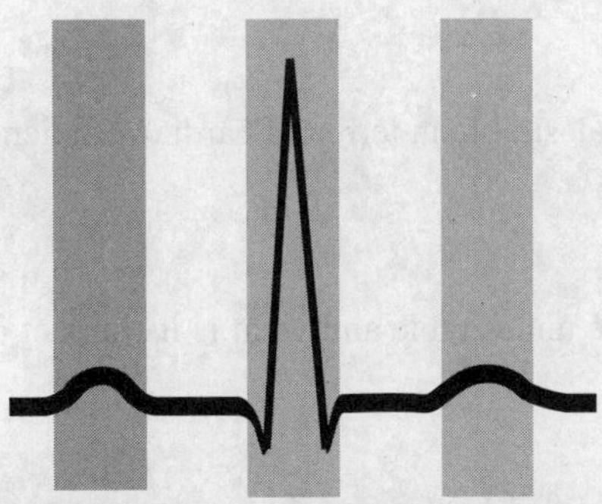

Copyright © 2027 by Elsevier, Inc. All rights are reserved, including those for text and data mining, AI training, and similar technologies.

36. Explain what is represented by each segment of the ECG tracing:

i. P wave:

ii. QRS complex:

iii. T wave:

37. Define cardiac dysrhythmia and explain how it affects cardiac output.

38. List at least three conditions in which cardiac arrhythmias occur.

39. Match the following definitions with the correct term:

i. heart rate greater than 350 beats per minute	i. cardioversion
ii. extra heartbeat arising in the ventricles	ii. bradycardia
iii. heart rate less than 60 beats per minute	iii. ectopic beat
iv. slowing or no transmission of impulses between atria and ventricles	iv. flutter
v. additional heartbeat originating in atria	v. fibrillation
vi. restoration of normal cardiac rhythm by electrical shock	vi. heart block
vii. heart rate between 160 and 350 beats per minute	vii. premature atrial contraction (PAC)
viii. extra beat originating outside the SA node	viii. premature ventricular contraction (PVC)
ix. heart rate between 100 and 160 beats per minute	ix. tachycardia

40. Why is a rapid (resting) heart rate undesirable in terms of cardiac efficiency?

41. Why is an excessively slow heart rate undesirable and what is its impact on systemic circulation?

Copyright © 2027 by Elsevier, Inc. All rights are reserved, including those for text and data mining, AI training, and similar technologies.

42. The drug groups identified in the accompanying chart are often prescribed alone or in combination to control dysrhythmias. Explain the action of each and how they would control or prevent arrhythmias. Also identify adverse effects and one example for each group.

Drug Group	Action and Effects	Adverse Effects	Example
β-Adrenergic blockers			
Calcium channel blockers			
Digitalis (cardiac glycosides)			

43. List two additional medications that might be prescribed for a patient with cardiac dysrhythmias and a history of atherosclerosis or angina and provide the rationale for each.

44. What type of pacemaker can be used by paramedics as an immediate life-saving treatment of an MI?

45. Why is it important to know whether a client has a pacemaker?

46. Define cardiac arrest and list a few potential causes.

HEART FAILURE

47. Identify **causes** of congestive heart failure.

48. Describe the **compensatory mechanisms** that are recruited in early heart failure to maintain cardiac output.

49. Explain the terms **"backup"** and **"forward"** effects in congestive heart failure and their physiological implications.

Copyright © 2027 by Elsevier, Inc. All rights are reserved,
including those for text and data mining, AI training, and similar technologies.

50. Complete the following chart comparing right-sided and left-sided heart failure:

	Right-Sided Heart Failure	Left-Sided Heart Failure
Cause		
Backup effects		
Forward effects		
Manifestations		

51. Explain why each of the following **manifestations** occurs with congestive heart failure:

i. splenomegaly:

ii. ascites:

iii. orthopnea:

iv. cough:

v. hemoptysis:

vi. distended neck veins:

vii. decreased urine output:

viii. nocturia:

ix. polycythemia:

Copyright © 2027 by Elsevier, Inc. All rights are reserved, including those for text and data mining, AI training, and similar technologies.

52. Many different **therapeutic interventions** are used in the treatment of congestive heart failure. Explain the rationale for each of the treatment measures listed below:

i. low sodium diet:

ii. low cholesterol diet:

iii. compression stockings:

iv. continuous oxygen therapy:

v. diuretics:

vi. potassium supplement:

vii. angiotensin-converting enzyme (ACE) inhibitors:

viii. digoxin:

ix. platelet inhibitor or anticoagulant:

x. sedative or antianxiety agent:

CONGENITAL HEART DEFECTS

53. List factors that may contribute to the **development** of congenital heart defects.

54. Define the following terms:

i. septal defect:

ii. valvular incompetence:

iii. regurgitation:

iv. prolapse:

v. stenosis:

vi. heart murmur:

Copyright © 2027 by Elsevier, Inc. All rights are reserved,
including those for text and data mining, AI training, and similar technologies.

55. How are most congenital heart defects **detected**?

56. Distinguish between a **"left-to-right shunt"** and a **"right-to-left shunt."** Describe the composition of systemic blood and explain the implications in each case.

57. Outline the signs and symptoms of large congenital heart defects in infants and children.

58. Explain the consequences of a **large ventricular septal defect**, including the complications that develop if the defect is not surgically corrected.

59. To understand the **consequences of a heart valve defect**, it is important to consider what is happening "behind" the valve (the **"backup" effect**), as well as what is happening "in front" of it (the **"forward" effect**). Complete the following chart comparing selected valve defects:

Defect	Backup Effects	Forward Effects	Manifestations
Mitral stenosis			
Mitral regurgitation			
Aortic stenosis			
Aortic regurgitation			
Pulmonary stenosis			
Pulmonary regurgitation			

60. Name two conditions that are usually associated with **heart murmurs**.

61. Describe the four defects that are present in **tetralogy of Fallot**. Outline the direction of blood flow or draw a diagram to illustrate blood direction. Describe the implications of altered blood flow.

Copyright © 2027 by Elsevier, Inc. All rights are reserved, including those for text and data mining, AI training, and similar technologies.

62. Describe **therapeutic interventions** used in the treatment of congenital heart defects.

63. A patient states that he previously had a heart murmur, but the defective valve was replaced with a prosthetic valve.

i. What medication will he be taking and why?

ii. What medications will he require if he is undergoing an invasive procedure such as dental surgery and why?

RHEUMATIC FEVER, RHEUMATIC HEART DISEASE, AND INFECTIVE ENDOCARDITIS

64. Identify the primary microorganism causing rheumatic fever and its role in the disease process.

65. Identify individuals who are at **high risk** for developing rheumatic fever.

66. Describe the **pathophysiology** of rheumatic fever, focusing on the immune response.

67. Describe the **manifestations** of rheumatic fever under the following headings:

i. general indication of systemic inflammation:

ii. pericarditis:

iii. myocarditis:

iv. endocarditis:

v. polyarthritis:

vi. skin manifestations:

vii. subcutaneous nodules:

viii. Sydenham's chorea:

68. Explain why endocarditis is the most serious complication of rheumatic fever.

Copyright © 2027 by Elsevier, Inc. All rights are reserved,
including those for text and data mining, AI training, and similar technologies.

69. Identify key measures used to **diagnose** rheumatic fever.

70. The **treatment of rheumatic fever** involves the use of several different types of drugs. Complete the following chart, identifying the effects of each type of medication as well as providing an example:

Medication	Effects	Example
Antibiotics		
Non-Steroidal Anti-Inflammatory Drugs (NSAIDs)		
Corticosteroids		
Antipyretic		
Antiarrhythmics		
Muscle relaxants		

71. Outline **other measures** (nonpharmaceuticals) used in the treatment of rheumatic fever.

72. Distinguish between **rheumatic fever** and **rheumatic heart disease**.

73. Which heart valve is **most commonly affected** by rheumatic heart disease?

74. Why is aspirin **(ASA)** often prescribed for individuals with a history of rheumatic heart disease?

75. Why are individuals with a history of rheumatic heart disease at an **increased risk** of developing **infective endocarditis**?

76. Why is **prophylactic antibiotic coverage** required before invasive procedures for individuals with rheumatic heart disease?

Copyright © 2027 by Elsevier, Inc. All rights are reserved, including those for text and data mining, AI training, and similar technologies.

77. Explain why someone with a **prosthetic heart valve** will still be required to take ASA (or some other platelet inhibitor or anticoagulant) for the rest of his or her life and why such a patient will still require antibiotic coverage before invasive procedures.

78. Differentiate between **subacute and acute infective endocarditis** (formerly known as *bacterial endocarditis*). Identify the microbial agents involved in each type.

79. Identify individuals who are at **high risk** for developing each type of infective endocarditis.

80. Outline the **pathophysiology** of infective endocarditis, focusing on vegetation formation.

81. Describe the **manifestations** and **complications** of infective endocarditis.

82. How is a **diagnosis** of infective endocarditis confirmed?

83. Describe the **treatment** for infective endocarditis, including duration and supportive measures.

84. Complete the following chart comparing rheumatic fever and infective endocarditis:

	Rheumatic Fever	Infective Endocarditis
Causative agent(s)		
Predisposing factors		
Manifestations and complications		
Antibiotic of choice		
Prophylactic antibiotic coverage?		

85. Name the possible causes of acute pericarditis and their impact on the pericardium.

Copyright © 2027 by Elsevier, Inc. All rights are reserved,
including those for text and data mining, AI training, and similar technologies.

HYPERTENSION

86. Define hypertension, including numerical blood pressure values and how age influences these criteria.

87. Differentiate between **essential** and **secondary** hypertension in terms of etiology and treatment.

88. What is meant by the term **"malignant hypertension"**?

89. Identify **predisposing factors** for hypertension, indicating those that are **modifiable**. Note that these parallel the risk factors for atherosclerosis and heart disease.

90. Describe the **pathophysiology** and **long-term complications** of undiagnosed or uncontrolled hypertension.

91. Explain why hypertension is often referred to as **"the silent killer."**

92. Describe **lifestyle and behavioral changes** that are recommended in the treatment of hypertension. Explain the rationale for each modification.

93. What is the **greatest problem** in the treatment of hypertension and strategies to address it?

ANTIHYPERTENSIVE MEDICATIONS

94. Complete the following chart comparing the most prescribed types of **antihypertensive agents**:

Type of Antihypertensive	Mechanism of Action and Effects	Adverse Effects	Examples
Diuretics			
ACE inhibitors			
Calcium channel blockers			
β-Adrenergic blockers			

Copyright © 2027 by Elsevier, Inc. All rights reserved, including those for text and data mining, AI training, and similar technologies.

95. Identify two **adverse effects** that are common to **all** antihypertensive medications.

96. List other medications that might be prescribed and state the rationale for each.

PERIPHERAL VASCULAR DISEASE

97. Describe the **general manifestations** of peripheral vascular disease (PVD).

98. Outline the various treatments used in treating PVD.

99. Define aortic **aneurysm**.

100. Identify the **causes** of aneurysms.

101. Describe the **complications** of aneurysms.

102. Identify factors that contribute to the **development of varicose veins**.

103. Describe the signs and symptoms of varicosities.

104. Differentiate between the clinical presentation of **thrombophlebitis** and **phlebothrombosis**.

105. Identify three factors that contribute to the **development of thrombophlebitis**.

Copyright © 2027 by Elsevier, Inc. All rights are reserved,
including those for text and data mining, AI training, and similar technologies.

106. Outline measures that could **decrease** the risk of developing thrombophlebitis.

107. What is a **pulmonary embolus**? Where did the blood clot probably originate?

SHOCK

108. Define **shock** and explain its impact on tissue perfusion.

109. Outline the **compensatory mechanisms** that are recruited as the blood pressure decreases.

110. Describe three **general manifestations** of shock, including the cause of each.

111. Identify the **potential complications** of shock and explain why each one occurs.

112. Outline general measures used in the **treatment** of shock.

113. Complete the following chart comparing the **different types of shock**:

Type of Shock	Etiology	Specific Manifestations	Specific Treatment
Hypovolemic or hemorrhagic			
Cardiogenic			
Anaphylactic			
Septic			
Neurogenic (syncope)			

Copyright © 2027 by Elsevier, Inc. All rights are reserved, including those for text and data mining, AI training, and similar technologies.

CONSOLIDATION

114. Identify the cardiovascular condition or conditions in which the following manifestations would be present:

i. ascites:

ii. positive Homan's sign:

iii. ECG changes:

iv. positive blood cultures:

v. claudication:

vi. hemoptysis:

vii. heart murmur:

viii. elevated cardiac enzymes:

ix. subcutaneous nodules:

x. pulmonary edema:

115. Identify the use or uses of the following drugs:

i. calcium channel blockers:

ii. nitroglycerine:

Copyright © 2027 by Elsevier, Inc. All rights are reserved,
including those for text and data mining, AI training, and similar technologies.

iii. penicillin:

iv. β-adrenergic blockers:

v. digoxin:

vi. diuretics:

vii. antidysrhythmics:

viii. ACE inhibitors:

116. Explain how **collateral circulation** can mitigate the effects of coronary artery disease and describe one method to promote its development.

117. Describe the role of the **renin-angiotensin-aldosterone system** in exacerbating congestive heart failure.

Copyright © 2027 by Elsevier, Inc. All rights reserved, including those for text and data mining, AI training, and similar technologies.

13 Respiratory System Disorders

1. Match the anatomical terms with the diagram of the respiratory system.

   Alveoli, Bronchiole, Diaphragm, Epiglottis, Heart, Larynx (voice box), Left lung, Left main bronchus, Lower respiratory system, Nasal cavity, Oral cavity, Pharynx, Pleura, Right lung, Right main bronchus, Tongue, Trachea, Upper respiratory system

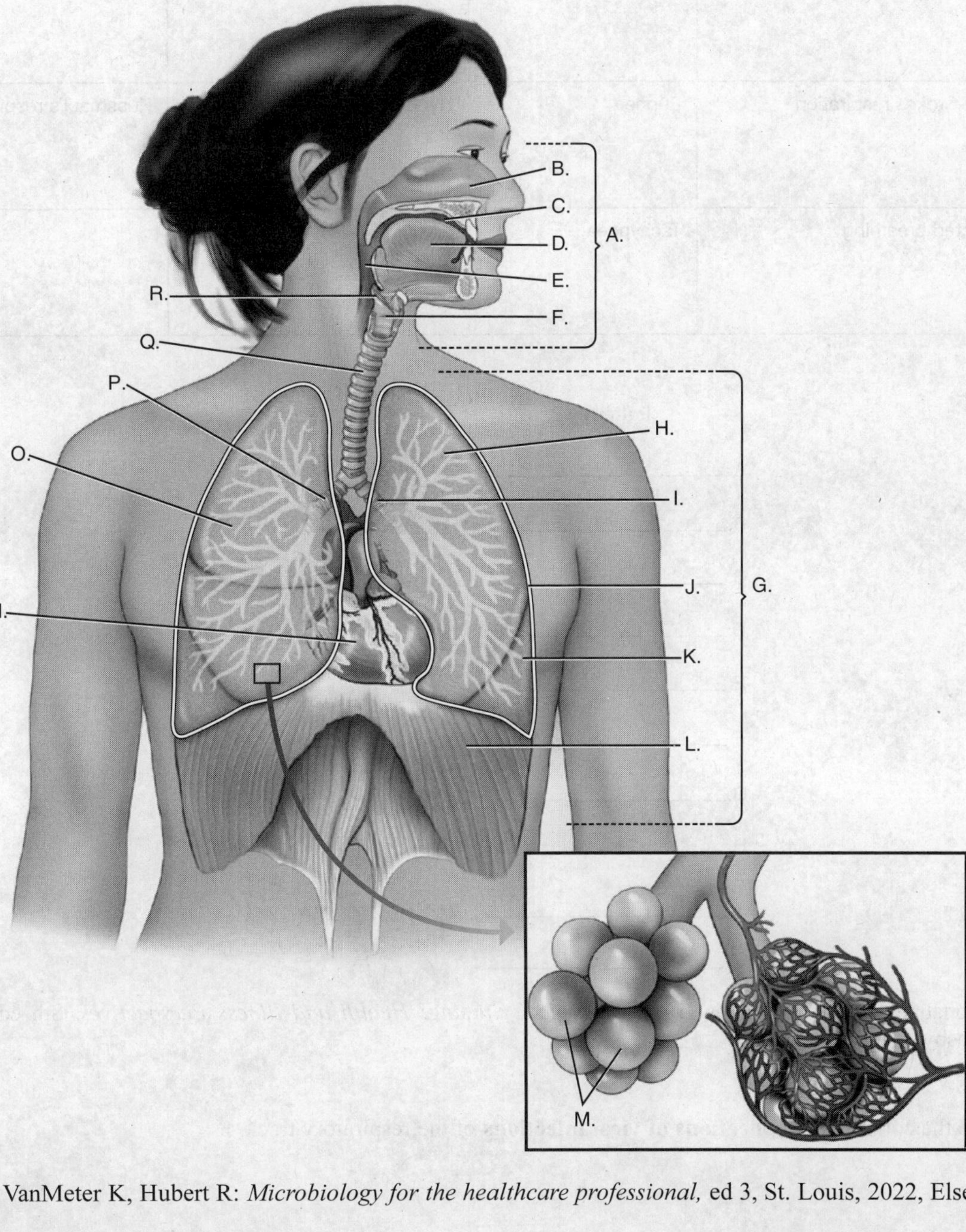

From VanMeter K, Hubert R: *Microbiology for the healthcare professional,* ed 3, St. Louis, 2022, Elsevier.

Copyright © 2027 by Elsevier, Inc. All rights are reserved, including those for text and data mining, AI training, and similar technologies.

A. ______________________
B. ______________________
C. ______________________
D. ______________________
E. ______________________
F. ______________________
G. ______________________
H. ______________________
I. ______________________
J. ______________________
K. ______________________
L. ______________________
M. ______________________
N. ______________________
O. ______________________
P. ______________________
Q. ______________________
R. ______________________

2. Match the pattern of breathing with the general manifestations of respiratory disease.

Apnea	Apneusis	Ataxic breathing	Bradypnea
Cheyne-Stokes respiration	Eupnea	Hyperpnea	Kussmaul's respiration
Obstructed breathing	Tachypnea		

Pattern

A. ______________________
B. ______________________
C. ______________________
D. ______________________
E. ______________________
F. ______________________
G. ______________________
H. ______________________
I. ______________________
J. ______________________

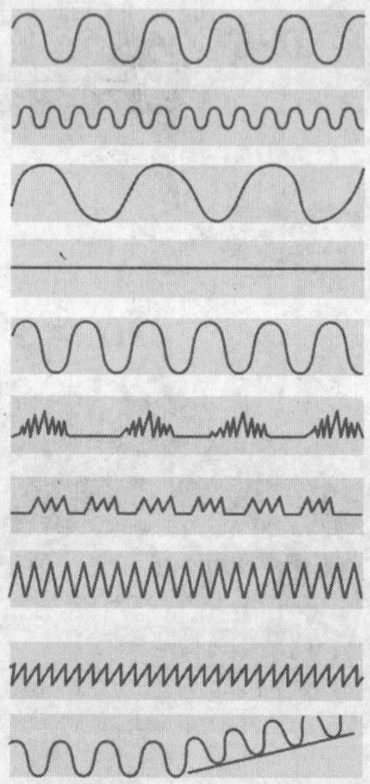

From Monahan FD, et al: *Phipps' Medical-Surgical Nursing: Health and Illness Perspectives,* 8th ed. St. Louis, 2007, Mosby.

3. Describe the common **complications of viral infections** of the respiratory tract.

Copyright © 2027 by Elsevier, Inc. All rights reserved, including those for text and data mining, AI training, and similar technologies.

4. Complete the following chart comparing and contrasting common childhood respiratory infections:

	Croup (Laryngotracheobronchitis)	Epiglottitis	Bronchiolitis
Usual age			
Cause			
Onset			
Pathology			
Significant signs and symptoms			
Treatment			

5. Complete the following chart comparing and contrasting selected types of **pneumonia**:

	Lobar Pneumonia	Bronchial Pneumonia	Interstitial Pneumonia
Causative agent			
Onset			
Distribution within lungs			
Pathophysiology			
Signs and symptoms			
Treatment			

Copyright © 2027 by Elsevier, Inc. All rights are reserved, including those for text and data mining, AI training, and similar technologies.

6. Briefly describe **Pneumocystis carinii pneumonia**. Identify individuals who are at high risk of contracting this type of pneumonia.

7. Name the microbial agent responsible for **severe acute respiratory syndrome (SARS)** and identify its mode of transmission.

8. Outline the **pathophysiology** of SARS.

9. Describe the signs and symptoms of SARS, including its effects on both blood gases and acid-base balance.

10. Identify the therapeutic interventions used in the treatment of SARS.

11. Identify the unique physiological characteristics of the virus that causes COVID-19.

12. Describe the two types of FDA approved tests to diagnose COVID-19.

13. Identify the therapeutic and/or prophylactic drugs for treatment of COVID-19.

14. Discuss the difficulties involved in controlling the spread of an infection when the causative agent is unidentified.

TUBERCULOSIS

15. Describe the characteristics of **Mycobacterium tuberculosis (TB)**.

16. Explain why it is difficult for host defensive cells to eradicate TB bacilli.

17. Identify individuals who are at **high risk** of contracting TB.

18. Describe the **pathophysiology** of TB, distinguishing between **primary** and **secondary infection**.

19. Describe the specific type of **lesion** that is associated with TB.

20. Outline the signs and symptoms of TB, distinguishing between those that occur with primary infection and those that develop with secondary infection or reinfection.

21. Briefly describe **miliary TB**.

Copyright © 2027 by Elsevier, Inc. All rights reserved, including those for text and data mining, AI training, and similar technologies.

22. How is a diagnosis of active (*i.e.,* infectious) TB **confirmed**?

23. What is a **Mantoux test**? What does a positive Mantoux indicate?

24. List **medications** used in the treatment of TB. Why is it necessary to take several different medications? What is the usual duration of drug therapy?

25. When will an individual who is taking TB medications become noncontagious? Explain why the drugs are prescribed for a longer period of time.

26. Individuals who are considered to be at high risk of contracting TB are routinely prescribed **TB prophylaxis**. Identify individuals who may require TB prophylaxis.

27. Identify the **medications** that are used for TB prophylaxis and the usual duration of treatment.

28. Describe measures that a **health care professional** should take to protect themselves against TB.

29. A client states that his last TB skin test was swollen and red. What additional information should be obtained from this individual?

30. An individual states that he had TB a number of years ago. What additional information should be obtained from this person?

CYSTIC FIBROSIS

31. What **type of disorder** is cystic fibrosis (CF)?

32. A baby is diagnosed with CF. Neither parent has this disorder. What are the genotypes of the parents? What is the probability that any of the baby's siblings will also have this disorder?

33. If an individual with CF had a child with an individual who was a carrier of CF, what is the probability that the child will have CF? What is the probability that they will be a carrier of CF?

34. Describe the **pathophysiology** of CF.

35. Outline the **manifestations** of CF.

36. Identify tools used in the **diagnosis** of CF.

Copyright © 2027 by Elsevier, Inc. All rights are reserved,
including those for text and data mining, AI training, and similar technologies.

37. Outline the treatments for CF.

38. What is the **life expectancy** of an individual with CF? What is the usual **cause of death**?

LUNG CANCER

39. Explain why the lungs are a frequent site of metastatic tumors.

40. List the **risk factors** for bronchogenic cancer.

41. Describe the **effects** of lung cancer.

42. Describe the signs and symptoms of lung cancer.

43. List treatments for lung cancer.

ASPIRATION

44. Define **aspiration**.

45. Identify individuals who are at **high risk** of aspiration.

46. Describe the effects of aspiration.

47. Identify common signs and symptoms of aspiration.

48. Describe the **Heimlich maneuver**.

ASTHMA

49. Define asthma.

50. Compare and contrast the two types of asthma (extrinsic and intrinsic).

51. Describe the **pathophysiology** of an asthmatic attack, identifying the three factors that interfere with normal ventilation.

52. Outline the **potential complications** of poorly controlled asthma.

53. Describe the progression of an **asthmatic attack**.

54. Identify **nonpharmacological measures** used in the treatment of asthma.

Copyright © 2027 by Elsevier, Inc. All rights are reserved, including those for text and data mining, AI training, and similar technologies.

55. Four types of **medications** are used in the control and treatment of asthma. Complete the following chart comparing and contrasting these drugs:

Drug Group	Action and Effects	Adverse Effects	Example and Route
Bronchodilators			
Corticosteroids			
Histamine release inhibitors			
Leukotriene receptor antagonists			

56. Identify which drug group can be used during an **acute asthmatic attack**.

57. An individual states he has asthma. What **additional information** should be obtained about his condition?

CHRONIC OBSTRUCTIVE PULMONARY DISEASE (COPD)

58. What is the **leading causative factor** for both emphysema and chronic bronchitis? Identify other **contributing factors** in the development of COPD.

59. Explain why **polycythemia** may develop in both advanced emphysema and chronic bronchitis.

60. Identify the underlying **pathology** involved in **emphysema**.

61. Loss of alveolar walls characteristically occurs with emphysema. Explain the consequences of this change.

62. Explain why individuals with emphysema are sometimes referred to as **"pink puffers."**

63. Outline the **complications** that develop with the progression of emphysema.

64. What impact does increased residual volume have on blood gases in advanced emphysema? How could this affect blood pH?

Copyright © 2027 by Elsevier, Inc. All rights are reserved,
including those for text and data mining, AI training, and similar technologies.

65. Explain how respiratory control mechanisms change as emphysema progresses.

66. What is meant by the term **"barrel chest"**? Explain why this condition develops in individuals with emphysema.

67. Outline the treatments for emphysema.

68. Describe the **pathophysiology of chronic bronchitis**.

69. Identify the **most significant symptom** of chronic bronchitis.

70. Explain why individuals with chronic bronchitis are sometimes referred to as **"blue bloaters."**

71. Describe the treatments for chronic bronchitis.

72. Complete the following chart comparing and contrasting selected chronic obstructive lung disorders:

	Asthma	Emphysema	Chronic Bronchitis
Etiology and predisposing factor			
Location			
Pathophysiology			
Signs and symptoms			
Complications			
Treatments			

Copyright © 2027 by Elsevier, Inc. All rights are reserved, including those for text and data mining, AI training, and similar technologies.

73. Define bronchiectasis and list two primary conditions/diseases that may cause it.

74. Define pneumoconiosis and state the usual treatment.

PULMONARY EDEMA

75. Identify the **causes** of pulmonary edema.

76. Describe the **pathophysiology** of pulmonary edema.

77. Describe the signs and symptoms of pulmonary edema.

78. Explain why the sputum of an individual with pulmonary edema might be frothy and possibly pink in color.

79. Explain why an individual with mild pulmonary edema will experience dyspnea when he is placed in a supine position (e.g., for dental treatment). What is the term used to describe this condition?

80. Outline the treatment of pulmonary edema, including medications that might be used.

PULMONARY EMBOLUS

81. Define **pulmonary embolus**.

82. Where do most pulmonary emboli **originate**? Identify other **potential sources** of pulmonary emboli.

83. Identify individuals who are at **high risk** for developing pulmonary emboli.

84. Describe the **pathophysiology** of a pulmonary embolus.

85. Identify the signs and symptoms of a pulmonary embolus.

86. What drugs may be used to **treat** pulmonary emboli?

EXPANSION DISORDERS

87. Explain the differences between **atelectasis** and **bronchiectasis**, including the etiologies, complications, and signs and symptoms.

88. Explain the differences between a **pleural effusion** and **pneumothorax**, including etiologies and signs and symptoms.

Copyright © 2027 by Elsevier, Inc. All rights are reserved,
including those for text and data mining, AI training, and similar technologies.

89. Explain what is meant by a **flail chest injury**.

90. Identify causes of **acute respiratory failure**.

91. Complete the following chart comparing and contrasting infant respiratory distress syndrome and adult respiratory distress syndrome:

	Infant Respiratory Distress Syndrome	Adult Respiratory Distress Syndrome
Etiology		
Pathophysiology		
Signs and symptoms		
Treatment		

92. Match each of the following definitions with the correct terms.

a. air in the pleural cavity — **i.pleural effusion**
b. abnormal widening of the bronchi — **ii.atelectasis**
c. excessive fluid in pleural cavity — **iii. pneumothorax**
d. chronic disorder resulting from continued exposure to irritating particles — **iv. bronchiectasis**
e. fungal infection of the lungs — **v.histoplasmosis**
f. collapse of a portion of the lung — **vi. pneumoconiosis**

CONSOLIDATION

93. For each of the following characteristics or definitions, identify the appropriate respiratory disorder or disorders in which they occur:

a. characterized by episodic bronchospasm:

b. causes orthopnea:

c. sputum often frothy and pink or blood-tinged:

d. loss of alveolar walls and lung elasticity:

Copyright © 2027 by Elsevier, Inc. All rights reserved, including those for text and data mining, AI training, and similar technologies.

e. caused by an acid-fast bacillus:

f. acute manifestations usually relieved by adrenergic agonists:

g. occurs most commonly in immunosuppressed individuals:

h. deficit of pancreatic digestive enzymes:

i. collapse of a lung or portion of a lung:

j. characterized by a constant productive cough:

k. a potential complication of thrombophlebitis in leg veins:

l. inadequate production of surfactant:

m. results from rib fractures:

n. defect in chloride ion transport in cell membranes:

o. causes malabsorption of nutrients:

p. may cause cavitation within lungs:

q. abnormal dilation of the bronchi:

r. accumulation of fluid in the pleural cavity:

s. characterized by caseation necrosis:

t. treated with leukotriene receptor antagonists:

Copyright © 2027 by Elsevier, Inc. All rights are reserved,
including those for text and data mining, AI training, and similar technologies.

14 Nervous System Disorders

ACUTE DISORDERS

1. Match the following terms with the anatomical parts of the brain and functional areas. The functional areas are indicated with a bold blank line on the figure.

(Central sulcus, Cerebellum, Frontal lobe, Lateral sulcus, Medulla, Motor cortex, Occipital lobe, Parietal lobe, Pons, Premotor cortex, Sensory cortex, Temporal lobe, Visual area, Visual association, Intellect Personality, Broca's Speech Area, Wernicke's Area, Auditory Area, Memory, Balance Equilibrium Coordination, Reticular Activating System, Vital Centers)

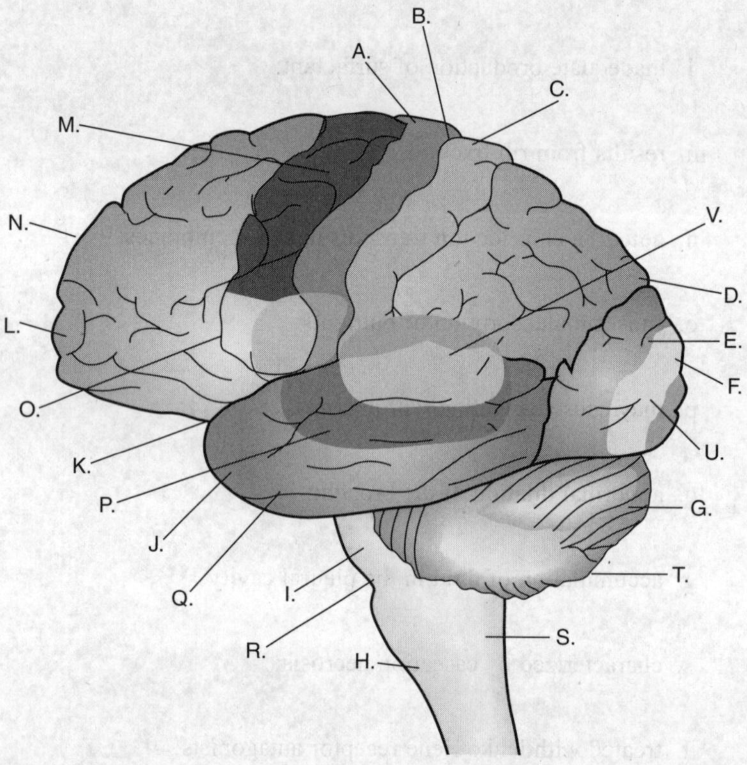

Anatomical Features

A. ____________________

B. ____________________

C. ____________________

D. ____________________

E. ____________________

F. ____________________

G. ____________________

H. ____________________

I. ____________________

J. ____________________

K. ____________________

L. ____________________

M. ____________________

Functional Features

N. ____________________

O. ____________________

P. ____________________

Q. ____________________

R. ____________________

S. ____________________

T. ____________________

U. ____________________

V. ____________________

Copyright © 2027 by Elsevier, Inc. All rights are reserved, including those for text and data mining, AI training, and similar technologies.

2. Name the meninges and the spaces between the layers.

3. What is the main function of the cerebrospinal fluid (CSF), and which structure forms the CSF?

4. Name the neurotransmitter that is acting at:

   i. the neuromuscular junction but also in the central nervous system:

   ii. preganglionic synapse of the autonomic nervous system:

   iii. postsynaptic synapses of the parasympathetic nervous system and the primary neurotransmitter at postsynaptic synapses of the sympathetic nervous system:

5. Describe the action of the sympathetic branch of the autonomic nervous system on the following:

   i. heart:

   ii. adrenal medulla:

   iii. respiratory system:

   iv. eye:

   v. digestive system function:

6. One of the early notable changes in individuals with acute brain disorders is a decreasing level of consciousness or responsiveness. Which areas of the brain are involved in the maintenance of consciousness?

7. Name the criteria that are generally used in the diagnosis of brain death and explain how this diagnosis is made.

8. Define aphasia and briefly describe the three main types, including areas of the brain affected.

9. Identify conditions that can lead to the development of **increased intracranial pressure**.

Copyright © 2027 by Elsevier, Inc. All rights are reserved, including those for text and data mining, AI training, and similar technologies.

10. Describe the **consequences** of increased intracranial pressure.

11. Identify the **manifestations** of increased intracranial pressure, explaining why each one occurs.

Tumors

12. Manifestations of brain tumors, whether they originate in the brain or are metastatic tumors, are primarily caused by their space-occupying effect and the replacement of normal tissue by tumor cells. Summarize the potential **generalized (*i.e.,* nonfocal) manifestations** of brain tumors.

Transient ischemic attacks and Cerebrovascular accidents

13. Define **transient ischemic attack (TIA)**.

14. Describe the **manifestations** of a TIA.

15. Explain the **significance** of TIAs.

16. Differentiate between a TIA and a stroke (cerebrovascular accident [CVA]).

17. List the risk factors for experiencing a CVA or stroke.

18. Describe the common **warning signs** of a stroke. Explain why they are often the same as the manifestations of a TIA.

19. Identify the three common **categories of CVA** or stroke, indicating which one occurs most commonly.

20. Describe the general **pathophysiology** of a CVA.

Copyright © 2027 by Elsevier, Inc. All rights are reserved, including those for text and data mining, AI training, and similar technologies.

21. Complete the following chart comparing and contrasting the three most common types of CVAs:

	Thrombus CVA	Embolus CVA	Hemorrhage CVA
Predisposing factors			
Onset			
Effects			
Immediate treatment			
Prognosis			

22. Identify the possible origins of **cerebral emboli**.

23. Explain why the **prognosis** for a hemorrhagic type stroke is worse than that for other types.

24. Describe the possible **manifestations** of a stroke under the following headings:

i. motor deficits:

ii. sensory deficits:

iii. speech deficits:

iv. cognitive and emotional manifestations:

25. Describe the **therapeutic interventions** used in the long-term treatment of an individual who has experienced a stroke (CVA), including medications.

Copyright © 2027 by Elsevier, Inc. All rights are reserved,
including those for text and data mining, AI training, and similar technologies.

26. An individual suffers a massive thrombus-type CVA involving the left frontal and parietal lobes. Describe the manifestations that they would probably experience.

Cerebral Aneurysms

27. What is a cerebral **aneurysm**? Include a description of its common locations and appearance.

28. Identify the most common factor that precipitates **rupture** of an aneurysm.

29. Describe **manifestations** of both an enlarging and a ruptured aneurysm.

Infections

30. Complete the following chart comparing and contrasting **meningitis** and **encephalitis**:

	Meningitis	Encephalitis
Causative agents		
Predisposing factors		
Pathophysiology		
Manifestations		
Treatment		

31. Identify the causative agent of shingles and describe the circumstances under which it typically manifests.

32. Describe the pathophysiology associated with Reye syndrome.

Copyright © 2027 by Elsevier, Inc. All rights are reserved, including those for text and data mining, AI training, and similar technologies.

Injuries

33. Briefly describe the following types of head injuries:

  i. concussion:

  ii. contusion:

  iii. linear fracture:

  iv. compound fracture:

  v. basilar fracture:

  vi. contrecoup injury:

34. Identify the location of the following hematomas:

  i. epidural:

  ii. subdural:

  iii. subarachnoid:

  iv. intracerebral:

35. Describe the **consequences and potential complications** of a head injury.

36. Describe the common **general manifestations** of head injuries.

37. Identify the common **causes** of **spinal cord injuries**.

Copyright © 2027 by Elsevier, Inc. All rights are reserved,
including those for text and data mining, AI training, and similar technologies.

38. Identify therapeutic interventions for the **treatment** of a head injury.

39. Outline the **consequences and potential complications** of a spinal cord injury.

40. Describe the potential **manifestations** of a spinal cord injury.

41. Identify the **therapeutic interventions** used in the treatment of spinal cord injuries.

42. Complete the following crossword puzzle:

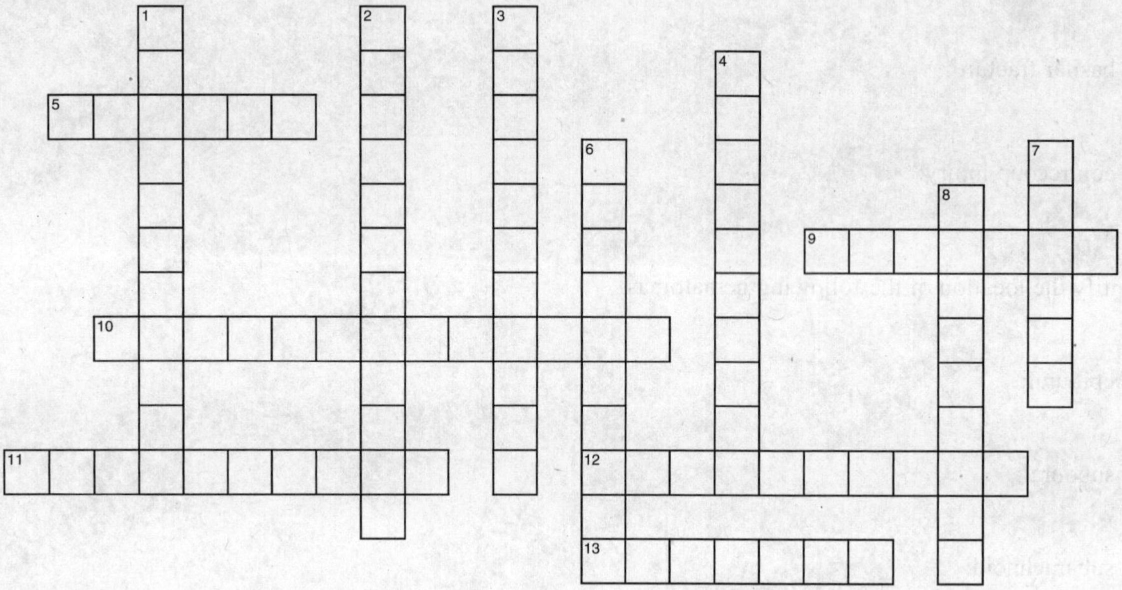

ACROSS

5. drooping eyelid
9. inability to recognize everyday objects
10. opposite side
11. difficulty pronouncing words
12. paralysis of lower half of body
13. inability to express or comprehend speech

DOWN

1. increased sensitivity to light
2. paralysis of all four limbs
3. same side
4. paralysis of one side of the body
6. loss of vision from the medial side of one eye and the lateral side of the other eye
7. brain tumor originating in neuroglial cells
8. bruising of the brain

Copyright © 2027 by Elsevier, Inc. All rights are reserved, including those for text and data mining, AI training, and similar technologies.

CONGENITAL NEUROLOGICAL DISORDERS

Hydrocephalus

43. Define **hydrocephalus**.

44. Identify the **causes** of hydrocephalus.

45. Outline the **pathophysiology** of hydrocephalus.

46. Distinguish between **noncommunicating** (obstructive) and **communicating** hydrocephalus.

47. Describe the signs and symptoms of hydrocephalus, differentiating between manifestations in infants and older children/adults.

48. What is the **treatment** for hydrocephalus?

Spina Bifida

49. Identify the **basic defect** involved in spina bifida.

50. Describe the three **types** of spina bifida and match those types to the diagrams.

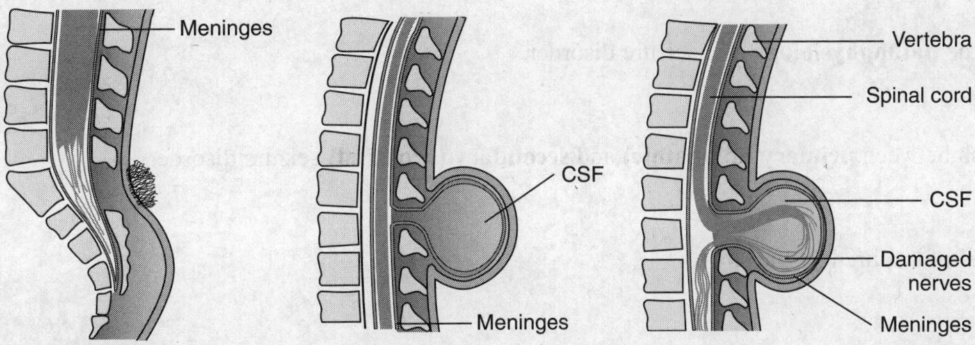

A.____________________ B.____________________ C.____________________

Copyright © 2027 by Elsevier, Inc. All rights are reserved, including those for text and data mining, AI training, and similar technologies.

51. How is spina bifida **diagnosed** prenatally?

52. List the possible **etiological factors** for spina bifida.

53. Describe the range of possible **signs and symptoms** of spina bifida.

54. Outline the **treatment** of spina bifida.

Cerebral Palsy

55. List the **causes** of cerebral palsy.

56. Describe the **pathophysiology** of cerebral palsy, emphasizing the nature and timing of the brain damage involved.

57. Describe the three major classifications of **motor disabilities** that occur with cerebral palsy.

58. Identify other possible **manifestations** of cerebral palsy.

59. Outline the **treatment** of cerebral palsy.

Seizure Disorders

60. Define **seizure**.

61. Describe the **pathophysiology** of a seizure disorder.

62. Distinguish between **primary (idiopathic)** and **secondary (acquired)** seizure disorders.

63. List **causes** of acquired seizures.

64. Differentiate between a **generalized seizure** and a **partial seizure**.

65. Describe an **absence**, or **petit mal, seizure**, including its typical clinical presentation and duration.

Copyright © 2027 by Elsevier, Inc. All rights are reserved, including those for text and data mining, AI training, and similar technologies.

66. What is meant by **prodromal signs**?

67. Define an **aura**, provide several examples, and explain its clinical significance.

68. Identify factors that might **precipitate a seizure** in an individual who suffers from epilepsy.

69. Describe a **tonic clonic (grand mal) seizure**. What is the typical **duration** of this type of seizure?

70. What are the **potential complications** of a seizure?

71. Outline the **emergency treatment** of a seizure.

72. Under what circumstances during or after a seizure is it necessary to seek emergency **medical assistance**?

73. Differentiate between a **simple partial** and a **complex partial seizure**.

74. Identify two major classes of **medications** prescribed to prevent seizures.

75. Describe the common and serious **adverse effects** associated with antiseizure medications

76. Define **status epilepticus** and identify the drugs typically used for its immediate treatment.

77. An individual states that he suffers from epilepsy. What **additional information** should you obtain before initiating treatment?

78. What measures should be taken to decrease the possibility of precipitating a seizure?

79. What diagnostic tests are used to determine the following?

  i. type and location of seizure:

  ii. structural abnormalities in the brain:

Copyright © 2027 by Elsevier, Inc. All rights are reserved,
including those for text and data mining, AI training, and similar technologies.

CHRONIC DEGENERATIVE DISORDERS

Multiple Sclerosis

80. Describe the characteristic pathological changes that occur in the central nervous system associated with multiple sclerosis (MS).

81. What is known about the **etiology** of MS?

82. Identify individuals who are at **high risk** for developing MS.

83. Describe how the characteristic lesions of MS affect nerve conduction.

84. What **components of the neurons** and which specific cells in the central nervous system are affected by MS?

85. How is MS **diagnosed**?

86. Describe the **manifestations** of MS, distinguishing between early and late symptoms.

87. Outline the **therapeutic interventions** used in the treatment of MS.

88. Explain the rationale for the use of corticosteroids and interferon in the treatment of MS.

Parkinson Disease

89. What is Parkinson disease?

90. State the underlying **pathological change** that occurs in Parkinson and the resulting neurochemical imbalance.

91. Describe the **manifestations** of Parkinson disease, distinguishing between early and later symptoms.

92. What drug group may cause drug-induced parkinsonism?

93. List drug groups that are used in the **treatment** of Parkinson disease.

Copyright © 2027 by Elsevier, Inc. All rights are reserved, including those for text and data mining, AI training, and similar technologies.

Amyotrophic lateral sclerosis, Myasthenia Gravis, and Huntington Disease

94. Amyotrophic lateral sclerosis (ALS), myasthenia gravis, and Huntington disease are all progressive neurological disorders that cause motor deficits. Complete the following chart comparing and contrasting these three conditions:

	ALS	Myasthenia Gravis	Huntington Disease
Etiology			
Pathophysiology			
Manifestations			
Treatment			
Prognosis			

Dementia

95. State several **causes** of dementia.

96. Outline the typical **pathophysiological** and structural changes that occur in the brain of an individual with Alzheimer disease.

97. List the **causes** of **Alzheimer disease.**

98. Identify the **signs and symptoms** of Alzheimer disease.

Copyright © 2027 by Elsevier, Inc. All rights are reserved,
including those for text and data mining, AI training, and similar technologies.

Mental Illness

99. Summarize the categories of **behavior** exhibited by individuals with **schizophrenia**.

100. Describe the **adverse effects** of **antipsychotic medications**.

101. Identify the major **classes of antidepressant drugs** and state an example of each.

Panic Disorder

102. Describe the signs and symptoms of panic disorder.

SPINAL CORD DISORDER

Herniated Disk

103. Describe the anatomical changes that occur in a herniated intervertebral disk.

104. What is the most serious **complication** of a herniated disk?

105. Identify the **most common site** of a herniated disk and describe the resulting **manifestations**.

106. Outline the **treatment** of a herniated lumbar disk.

Consolidation

107. A client has a history of **cognitive impairment**. What **additional information** should you try to obtain?

108. Identify how treatment should be modified for an individual with a history of cognitive impairment.

109. For each of the following pathological findings/characteristics, identify the condition or conditions in which they occur:

    i. loss of myelin in the central nervous system (CNS):

    ii. impairment of receptors at neuromuscular junctions:

Copyright © 2027 by Elsevier, Inc. All rights are reserved, including those for text and data mining, AI training, and similar technologies.

iii. reduced function of the basal ganglia (nuclei):

iv. development of neurofibrillary tangles:

v. decreased dopamine synthesis:

vi. depletion of gamma-aminobutyric acid:

vii. degeneration of both upper and lower motor neurons:

viii. an autosomal dominant disorder:

ix. an autoimmune disorder:

x. rigidity and difficulty in initiating movements:

xi. development of plaques in the brain:

xii. decreased levels of acetylcholine in the CNS:

xiii. treated with levodopa:

xiv. treated with donepezil:

xv. caused by infection by a prion:

Copyright © 2027 by Elsevier, Inc. All rights are reserved,
including those for text and data mining, AI training, and similar technologies.

15 Disorders of the Eye, Ear, and Other Sensory Organs

EYE

1. Match the structures of the eye with the terms.

Anterior chamber, Canal of Schlemm, Central retinal artery and vein, Choroid, Ciliary muscle, Conjunctiva, Cornea, Fovea centralis, Iris, Lateral rectus muscle, Lens, Medial rectus muscle, Meninges, Optic disc ("blind spot"), Optic nerve, Posterior cavity (vitreous humor), Posterior chamber, Pupil, Retina, Retinal artery, Retinal vein, Sclera, Suspensory ligament

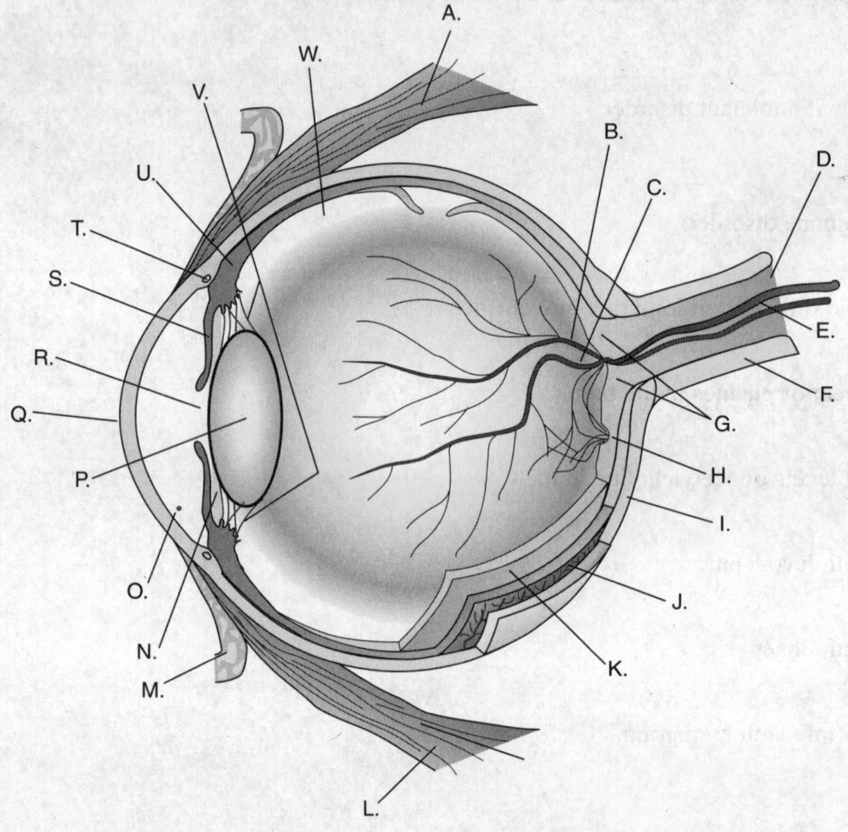

A. ____________________ I. ____________________ Q. ____________________
B. ____________________ J. ____________________ R. ____________________
C. ____________________ K. ____________________ S. ____________________
D. ____________________ L. ____________________ T. ____________________
E. ____________________ M. ____________________ U. ____________________
F. ____________________ N. ____________________ V. ____________________
G. ____________________ O. ____________________ W. ____________________
H. ____________________ P. ____________________

Copyright © 2027 by Elsevier, Inc. All rights reserved, including those for text and data mining, AI training, and similar technologies.

2. Explain the use of the following basic diagnostic tests:

   i. Snellen chart:

   ii. visual field test:

   iii. tonometry:

   iv. ophthalmoscope:

   v. gonioscopy:

3. Define the following functional defects associated with the eye:

   i. myopia:

   ii. hyperopia:

   iii. presbyopia:

   iv. astigmatism:

   v. diplopia:

4. Describe the following eye infections, including the causative agent(s):

   i. stye:

   ii. conjunctivitis:

   iii. trachoma:

   iv. keratitis:

5. State the **basic pathology** involved in glaucoma.

6. Differentiate between **narrow-angle** and **wide-angle** glaucoma.

Copyright © 2027 by Elsevier, Inc. All rights are reserved,
including those for text and data mining, AI training, and similar technologies.

7. Identify individuals who are at **increased risk** of developing glaucoma.

8. List the **manifestations** of glaucoma.

9. Outline the therapeutic interventions used in the **treatment** of glaucoma.

10. Complete the following chart comparing common ocular problems.

	Cataract	Macular Degeneration	Retinal Detachment
Etiology			
Pathology			
Effect on vision			
Treatment			

11. List and briefly describe the treatments for both types of age-related macular degeneration (ARMD).

12. For each of the following pathological findings/characteristics, identify the condition(s) in which they occur:

i. characterized by clouding of the ocular lens:

ii. characterized by degeneration of the fovea centralis:

iii. treated with cholinergic eye drops:

iv. characterized by loss of central vision:

v. appearances of "halos" around lights:

vi. increased intraocular pressure:

Copyright © 2027 by Elsevier, Inc. All rights reserved, including those for text and data mining, AI training, and similar technologies.

EAR

13. Match the terms with the structures of the ear shown in the diagram.

Auditory (eustachian) tube, Auditory nerve (VIII), Auditory ossicles, Cochlea containing organ of Corti, Cochlear nerve, External auditory canal, External ear, Incus, Inner ear, Malleus, Middle ear, Oval window, Pinna, Semicircular canals, Stapes, Temporal bone, Tympanic membrane, Vestibular, Vestibule

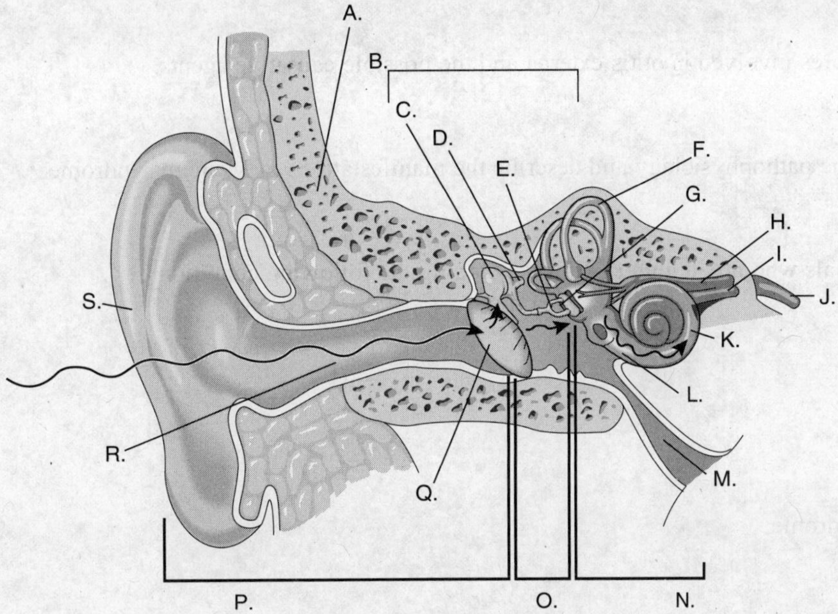

A. ______________________

B. ______________________

C. ______________________

D. ______________________

E. ______________________

F. ______________________

G. ______________________

H. ______________________

I. ______________________

J. ______________________

K. ______________________

L. ______________________

M. ______________________

N. ______________________

O. ______________________

P. ______________________

Q. ______________________

R. ______________________

S. ______________________

Copyright © 2027 by Elsevier, Inc. All rights are reserved,
including those for text and data mining, AI training, and similar technologies.

14. Differentiate between conduction deafness and sensorineural deafness, and state several examples of each type.

15. Define otitis media and common microorganisms causing the infection.

16. Discuss the treatment options for otitis media.

17. Name the structures involved in otitis externa and the possible causative agents.

18. Briefly outline the pathophysiology and describe the manifestations of Ménière syndrome.

19. Identify individuals who are at high risk for developing the following conditions:

    i. otitis media:

    ii. otitis externa:

    iii. Ménière syndrome:

Copyright © 2027 by Elsevier, Inc. All rights reserved, including those for text and data mining, AI training, and similar technologies.

16 Endocrine System Disorders

1. Match the following terms with the endocrine glands depicted in the diagram.

   Adrenal gland, Kidney, Ovary in female, Pancreas, Parathyroid glands on posterior thyroid, Pineal gland, Pituitary gland, Testes in male, Thymus, Thyroid gland

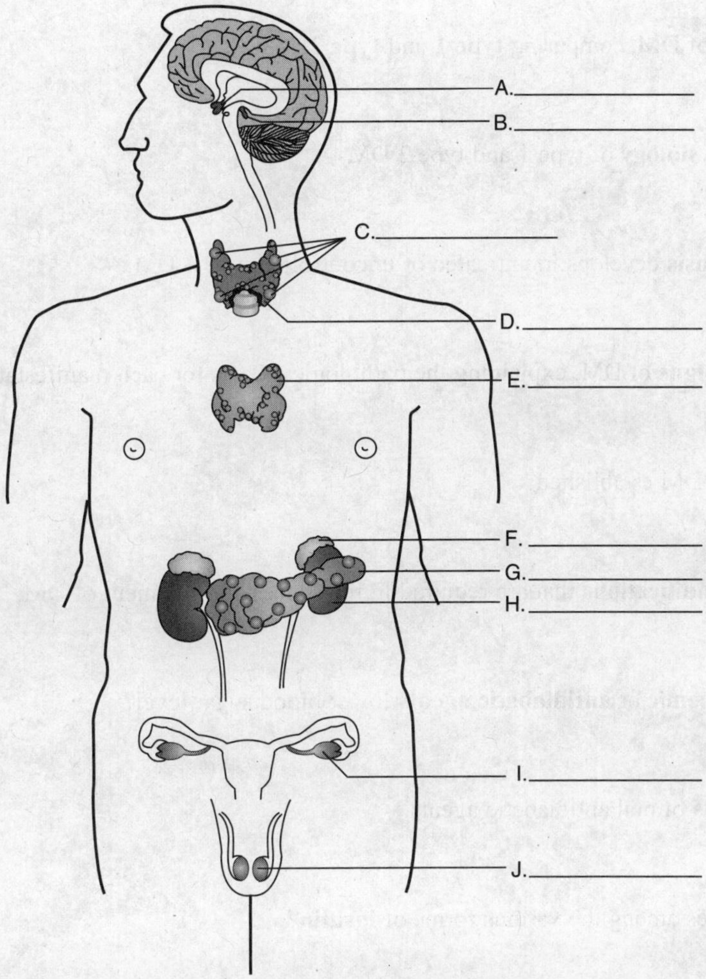

A. ______________________ F. ______________________
B. ______________________ G. ______________________
C. ______________________ H. ______________________
D. ______________________ I. ______________________
E. ______________________ J. ______________________

2. Define hormones and their classification; give an example of each type.

3. What is the major mechanism that controls hormone levels in the blood?

Copyright © 2027 by Elsevier, Inc. All rights are reserved, including those for text and data mining, AI training, and similar technologies.

4. Describe the two primary categories of hormonal imbalance that lead to endocrine disorders.

5. What tests are commonly used to check the serum level of a hormone?

DIABETES MELLITUS

6. List the **predisposing factors** for developing diabetes mellitus (DM).

7. Describe the **etiology** of DM, comparing **type 1** and **type 2**.

8. Describe the **pathophysiology** of type 1 and type 2 DM.

9. Explain why **ketoacidosis** develops in untreated or uncontrolled type 1 DM.

10. Identify the **warning signs** of DM, explaining the pathological basis for each manifestation.

11. How is a **diagnosis** of DM established?

12. Outline the **dietary modifications** that are required in the successful treatment of DM.

13. How do **oral hypoglycemic** or **antidiabetic agents** lower blood sugar level?

14. List the **adverse effects** of oral antidiabetic agents.

15. What are the differences among the various forms of **insulin**?

16. How is insulin administered?

17. Identify factors that could precipitate a **hypoglycemic** or **insulin reaction**.

18. Identify measures that could minimize the chances of a diabetic individual experiencing a hypoglycemic reaction.

Copyright © 2027 by Elsevier, Inc. All rights are reserved, including those for text and data mining, AI training, and similar technologies.

19. Distinguish between **microangiopathy** and **macroangiopathy**, including the consequences of each.

20. Explain what is meant by **peripheral neuropathy caused by diabetes**. Identify the causes and complications of diabetic neuropathy.

21. Explain why individuals with diabetes are considered to be at high risk for developing serious tissue trauma and **infections**.

22. Identify the **types of infections** that commonly occur in individuals with poorly regulated DM.

23. Explain why there may be **delayed healing** in an individual with DM.

24. What is **gestational diabetes**?

25. Complete the following chart comparing and contrasting the two **acute complications** that may occur in an individual who has diabetes:

	Hypoglycemic Shock	Ketoacidosis
Other names		
Cause		
Precipitating factors		
Speed of onset		
Manifestations		
Emergency treatment		
Speed of response to emergency treatment		
Prevention		

Copyright © 2027 by Elsevier, Inc. All rights are reserved,
including those for text and data mining, AI training, and similar technologies.

26. Complete the following chart comparing and contrasting type 1 and type 2 DM:

	Type 1	Type 2
Percentage of individuals with DM		
Age at onset		
Speed of onset of symptoms		
Family history		
Body build (BMI)		
Autoantibodies to beta cells?		
Insulin receptor defects		
Severity of manifestations		
Stability (*i.e.,* maintenance of normal blood glucose)		
Frequency of complications		
Occurrence of ketoacidosis		
Frequency of hypoglycemia		
Treatment with insulin		
Treatment with oral hypoglycemics		

Copyright © 2027 by Elsevier, Inc. All rights are reserved, including those for text and data mining, AI training, and similar technologies.

PARATHYROID DISORDERS

27. Identify the causes of hypoparathyroidism and hyperparathyroidism.

28. Identify the **consequences** of **hypoparathyroidism**.

29. Identify the **consequences** of **hyperparathyroidism**.

ACROMEGALY

30. State the **etiology** of acromegaly.

31. Outline the **manifestations** and **complications** of acromegaly.

ANTIDIURETIC HORMONE

32. Differentiate between diabetes insipidus and DM.

THYROID DISORDERS

33. What is a **goiter**? State the **etiology** of a goiter.

Copyright © 2027 by Elsevier, Inc. All rights are reserved, including those for text and data mining, AI training, and similar technologies.

34. Complete the following chart comparing and contrasting **hyperthyroidism** and **hypothyroidism**:

	Hyperthyroidism	Hypothyroidism
Forms		
Etiology		
Serum T3 and T4 levels		
Metabolic rate		
Nervous system effects		
Cardiovascular effects		
Respiratory effects		
Skeletal effects		
Muscular effects		
Skin and hair		
Temperature tolerance		
Eyes		
BMI		
Presence of goiter		
Treatment		

Copyright © 2027 by Elsevier, Inc. All rights are reserved, including those for text and data mining, AI training, and similar technologies.

ADRENAL DISORDERS

35. Complete the following chart comparing and contrasting **Cushing syndrome** and **Addison disease**:

	Cushing Syndrome	**Addison Disease**
Etiology		
Physical appearance		
Fluid and electrolytes		
Blood pressure		
Blood sugar		
Musculoskeletal effects		
Inflammatory response		
Immune response		
Response to stress		
Treatment		

36. Individuals with Cushing syndrome may be prescribed prophylactic antibacterial drugs before invasive procedures such as dental surgery. Explain the rationale for this.

Copyright © 2027 by Elsevier, Inc. All rights are reserved,
including those for text and data mining, AI training, and similar technologies.

MULTIPLE ENDOCRINE NEOPLASIA TYPE I

37. Describe the manifestations of multiple endocrine neoplasia type I.

CONSOLIDATION

38. For each of the following disorders, identify the etiology (*i.e.,* hyposecretion or hypersecretion of a specific hormone):

   i. Graves disease:

   ii. gigantism:

   iii. myxedema:

   iv. diabetes insipidus:

   v. acromegaly:

   vi. Cushing syndrome:

   vii. dwarfism:

   viii. DM:

   ix. Addison disease:

   x. cretinism:

39. For each of the following characteristics, identify the endocrine disorder or disorders in which it occurs:

   i. hyperglycemia:

   ii. increased basal metabolic rate:

   iii. increased susceptibility to infection:

   iv. intolerance to cold:

   v. development of osteoporosis or decreased bone density:

Copyright © 2027 by Elsevier, Inc. All rights are reserved, including those for text and data mining, AI training, and similar technologies.

vi. intellectual disability:

vii. predisposition to renal calculi:

viii. hypotension:

ix. impaired physical growth:

x. hyperpigmentation of the skin and oral mucosa:

xi. autoimmunity:

xii. development of peripheral edema:

xiii. development of exophthalmos:

xiv. bradycardia:

xv. delayed clotting:

xvi. poor healing:

xvii. poor response to stress:

xviii. development or exacerbation of hypertension:

xix. weight loss:

xx. presence of a goiter:

xxi. enlarged hands and feet:

xxii. tachycardia and palpitations:

xxiii. hyponatremia:

xxiv. hypocalcemia:

Copyright © 2027 by Elsevier, Inc. All rights are reserved,
including those for text and data mining, AI training, and similar technologies.

17 Digestive System Disorders

1. Match the following terms with the organs/structures of the digestive system depicted in the diagram.

   Anus, Appendix, Ascending colon, Cardiac sphincter, Cecum, Common bile duct, Descending colon, Diaphragm, Duodenal papilla, Duodenum, Esophagus, Gallbladder, Hard palate, Ileocecal valve, Ileum, Jejunum, Large intestine, Liver, Mouth, Oropharynx, Pancreas, Parotid salivary gland, Pyloric sphincter, Rectum, Sigmoid colon, Stomach, Sublingual salivary gland, Submandibular salivary gland, Tongue, Tooth, Trachea, Transverse colon

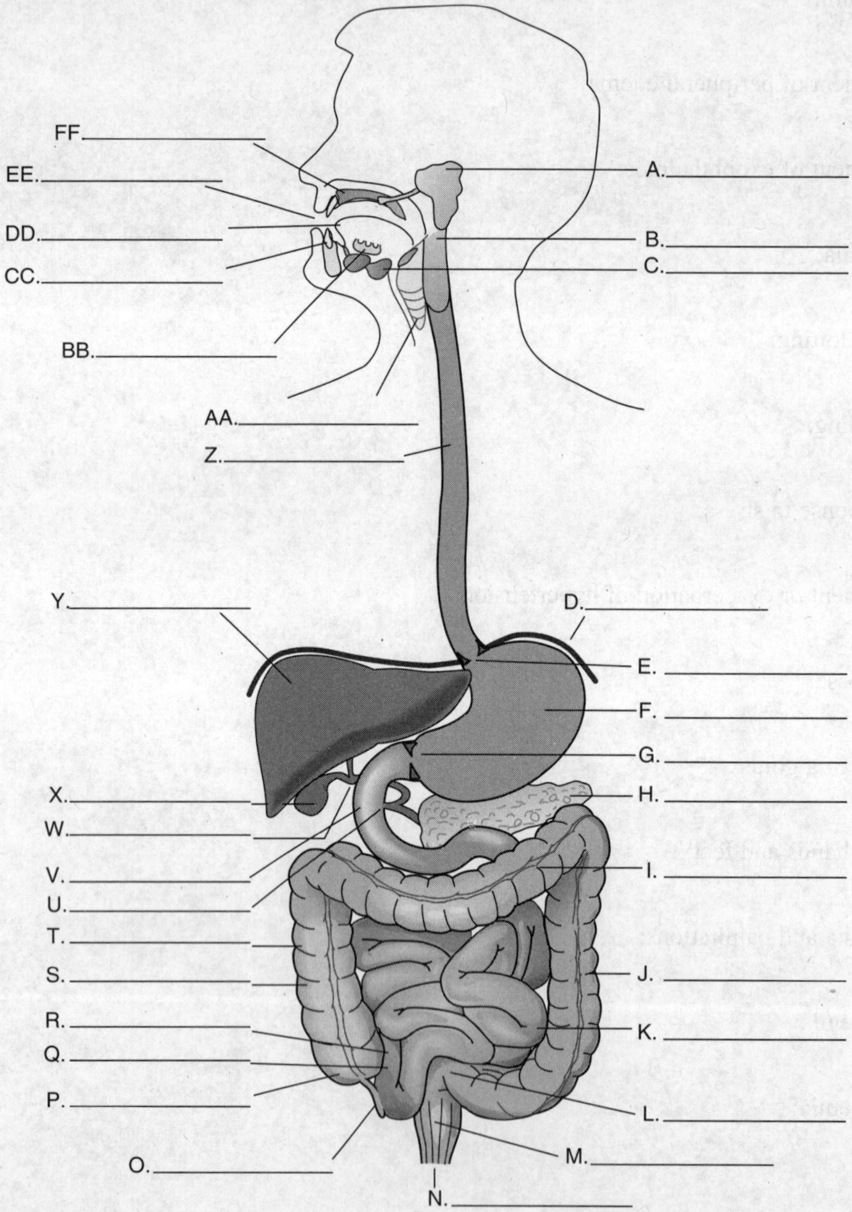

Copyright © 2027 by Elsevier, Inc. All rights are reserved, including those for text and data mining, AI training, and similar technologies.

2. Match the following definitions with the correct term:

a) drug used to decrease nausea and vomiting	i) **steatorrhea**
b) formation of gallstones	ii) **melena**
c) greasy, loose stools	iii) **dysphagia**
d) loss of appetite	iv) **antiemetic**
e) opportunistic oral fungal infection	v) **anorexia**
f) outpouching of the mucosa in colon	vi) **hematemesis**
g) tarry stools caused by bleeding	vii) **impaction**
h) difficulty swallowing	viii) **candidiasis**
i) inflammation of tissue surrounding the teeth	ix) **gingivitis**
j) retention of feces	x) **cholelithiasis**
k) vomit containing blood	xi) **diverticulum**

3. Identify six causes of vomiting, and state an example of each.

4. Outline measures that are used to decrease vomiting.

5. Identify nine causes of constipation.

6. What dietary modifications could help prevent chronic constipation?

Copyright © 2027 by Elsevier, Inc. All rights are reserved, including those for text and data mining, AI training, and similar technologies.

7. Identify the causes of **dysphagia** depicted in the diagrams.

Achalasia; Compression; Congenital atresia; Congenital tracheoesophageal; Diverticulum; Fibrosis; Neurological damage to cranial nerves V, VII, IX, X, and XII

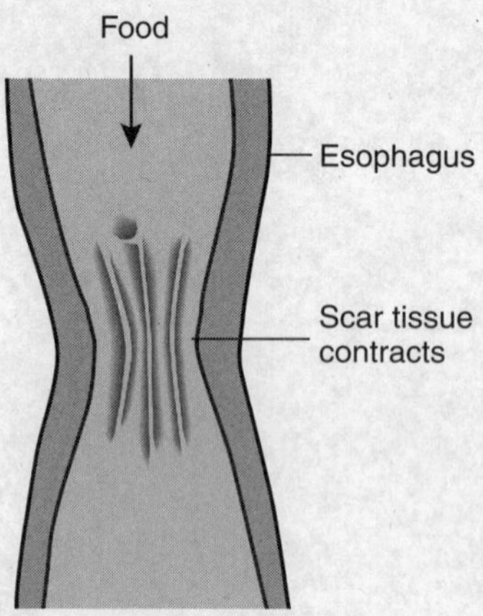

A. ____________

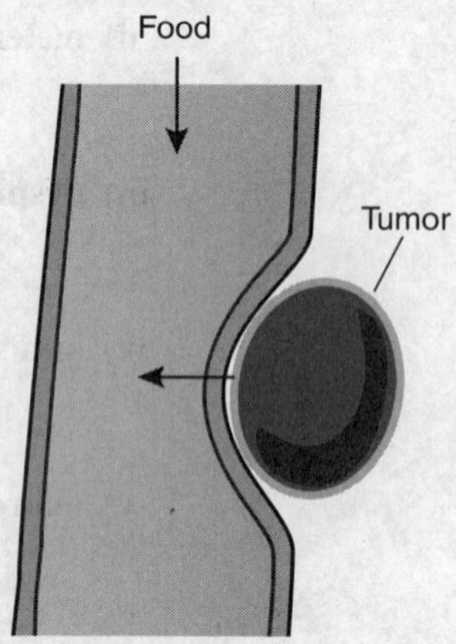

B. ____________

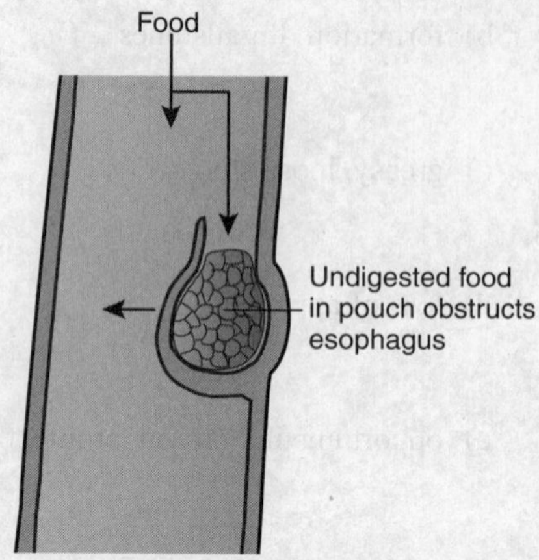

C. ____________

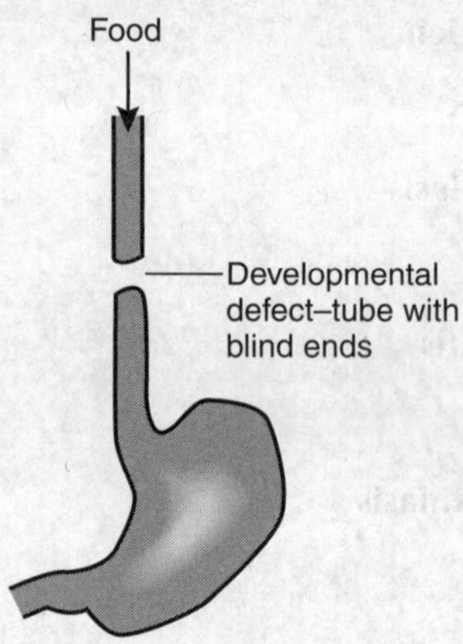

D. ____________

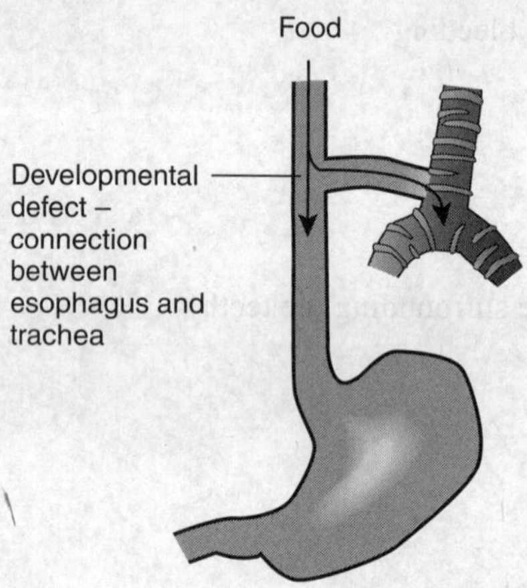

E. ____________

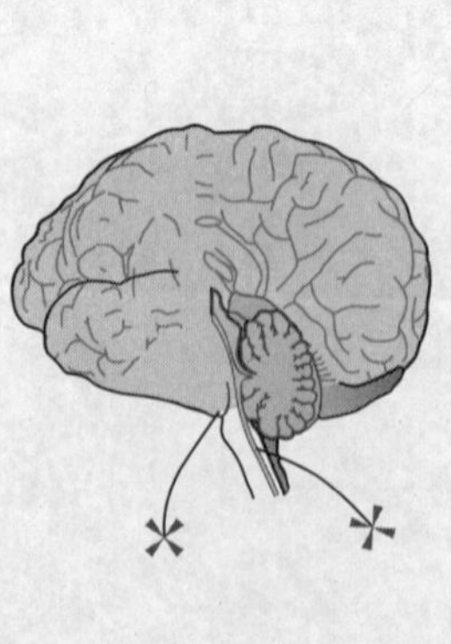

F. ____________

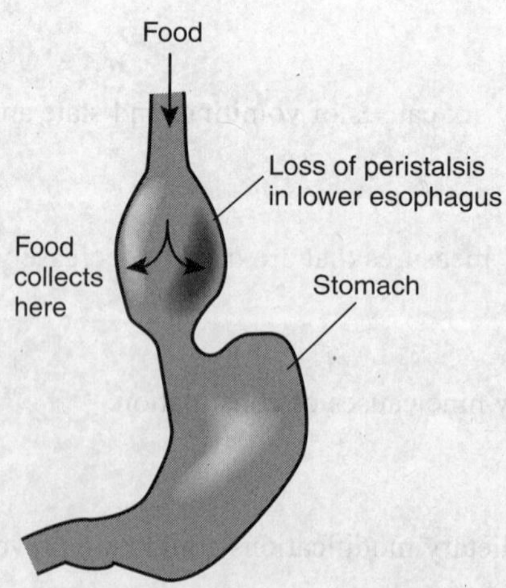

G. ____________

Copyright © 2027 by Elsevier, Inc. All rights are reserved, including those for text and data mining, AI training, and similar technologies.

8. Describe a **hiatal hernia**.

9. Describe the signs and symptoms of a hiatal hernia.

10. Outline helpful measures to reduce the discomfort of hiatal hernias by decreasing lower esophageal sphincter pressure.

11. What is **gastroesophageal reflux disease (GERD)**? Describe the **etiology** of GERD.

12. What types of medications are used in the treatment of GERD?

13. Distinguish between acute gastritis and acute gastroenteritis.

14. Differentiate between acute gastritis and chronic gastritis in relation to etiology and signs and symptoms.

15. Complete the following chart comparing and contrasting selected types of **food poisoning**:

Pathogen	Source	Incubation	Signs and Symptoms
Staphylococcus aureus			
Escherichia coli (*E. coli*, "traveler's diarrhea," or "hamburger disease")			
Salmonella			
Clostridium botulinum			

16. List and briefly describe the five forms of intestinal disease caused by an *E. coli* infection.

ULCERS

17. State the **locations** where peptic ulcers occur.

Copyright © 2027 by Elsevier, Inc. All rights are reserved,
including those for text and data mining, AI training, and similar technologies.

18. Identify **factors** that contribute to the development of peptic ulcers.

19. Describe the **pathophysiology** of peptic ulcers.

20. Outline the **potential complications** that may occur with peptic ulcers.

21. Describe the signs and symptoms of peptic ulcers.

22. Identify the treatment for simple peptic ulcers.

CANCER

23. Complete the following chart comparing and contrasting **cancer** of the gastrointestinal tract and accessory organs:

	Etiology	Pathophysiology	Symptoms and Complications	Treatment
Esophagus				
Stomach				
Liver				
Pancreas				
Colorectal				

GALLBLADDER DISEASE

24. Identify individuals who are considered **high risk** for developing **gallstones**.

25. Describe the **signs and symptoms of gallstones**.

Copyright © 2027 by Elsevier, Inc. All rights reserved, including those for text and data mining, AI training, and similar technologies.

LIVER DISEASE

26. State the three groups of disorders that may cause **jaundice**, and state examples of each.

27. Identify **causes** of **nonviral hepatitis**.

28. Complete the following chart comparing and contrasting the most common types of **viral hepatitis**:

	Hepatitis A	Hepatitis B	Hepatitis C
Causative agent			
Transmission			
High-risk groups			
Age			
Incubation period			
Duration of signs and symptoms			
Carrier state present/absent			
Complications			
Serological markers			
Medications			
Immunoglobulin			
Vaccine			

Copyright © 2027 by Elsevier, Inc. All rights are reserved, including those for text and data mining, AI training, and similar technologies.

29. Explain what is meant by the **"fecal-oral"** route of transmission. State several examples of how infections can be spread this way.

30. **Hepatitis D** occurs only in individuals who also have hepatitis B. Explain why.

31. How can **hepatitis D** infection be detected if the person also has hepatitis B?

32. How is **hepatitis E** contracted?

33. The signs and symptoms of all types of hepatitis are remarkably similar. What varies is the onset, severity, and duration of symptoms. Describe the **general** signs and symptoms of hepatitis.

34. Explain why it is often very difficult to track infection sources for those individuals with hepatitis B.

35. Define **cirrhosis**.

36. Identify **causes of cirrhosis**.

37. Describe the **pathophysiology** of cirrhosis.

38. Identify the **liver functions** that are lost or impaired with cirrhosis.

39. Describe the signs and symptoms that are a consequence of the losses identified in the previous question.

40. Explain what is meant by **portal hypertension** and how it develops.

41. Describe the **complications** that develop as a consequence of portal hypertension.

42. Outline the interventions for cirrhosis.

PANCREATITIS

43. Identify the **causes** of acute pancreatitis.

Copyright © 2027 by Elsevier, Inc. All rights are reserved, including those for text and data mining, AI training, and similar technologies.

44. Describe the **pathophysiology** of acute pancreatitis.

45. Identify the signs and symptoms of pancreatitis.

46. Outline the **treatment** of pancreatitis.

INTESTINAL DISORDERS

47. What is **celiac disease**?

48. Briefly describe the **pathophysiology** of celiac disease.

49. What are the characteristic signs and symptoms of malabsorption syndromes?

50. Outline the **treatment** of celiac disease.

51. Explain what is meant by **chronic inflammatory bowel disease**.

52. Complete the following chart comparing and contrasting Crohn disease and ulcerative colitis:

	Crohn Disease	**Ulcerative Colitis**
Individuals at high risk		
Etiology		
Location of lesions		
Characteristics of lesions		
Complications		
Signs and symptoms		

Copyright © 2027 by Elsevier, Inc. All rights are reserved,
including those for text and data mining, AI training, and similar technologies.

53. Describe the treatments for inflammatory bowel disease.

54. Describe the **pathophysiology** of appendicitis.

55. Outline the signs and symptoms of acute appendicitis.

56. List the methods to diagnose appendicitis.

57. Briefly describe the **pathophysiology** and a **complication** of diverticulitis.

58. List the **warning signs** of **colorectal cancer**.

59. Identify tools to diagnose colorectal cancer.

Copyright © 2027 by Elsevier, Inc. All rights are reserved, including those for text and data mining, AI training, and similar technologies.

60. Identify the **causes** of **intestinal obstruction** depicted in the diagrams.

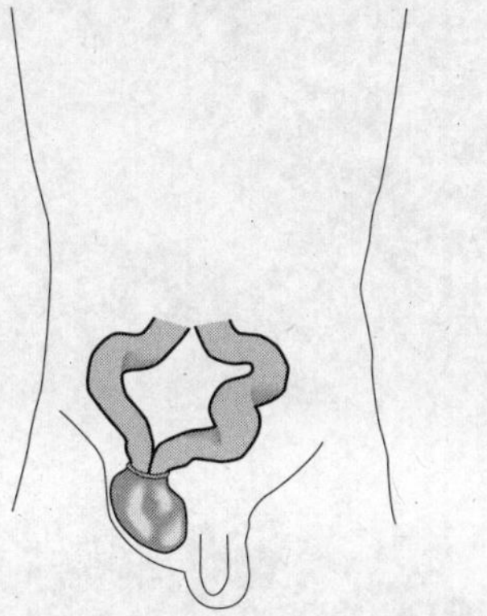

A. ______________________

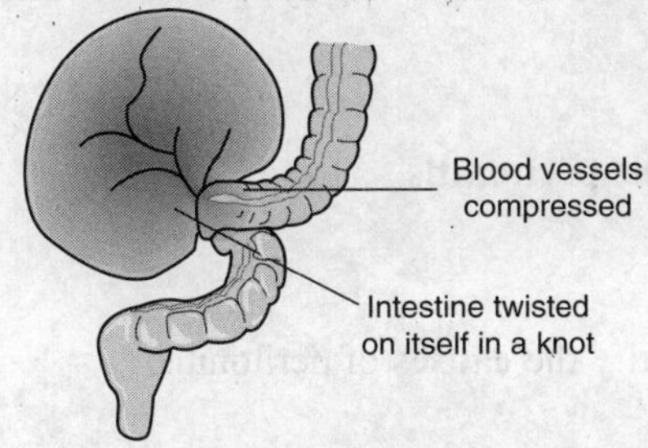

B. ______________________

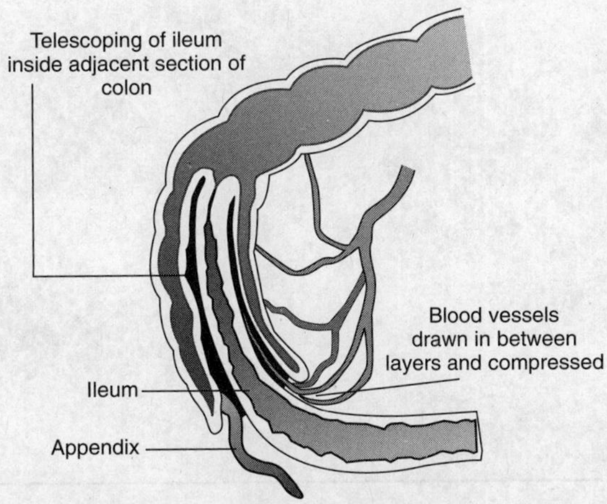

C. ______________________

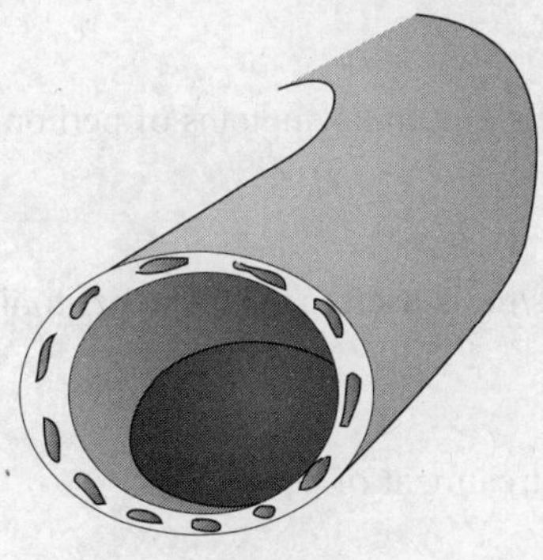

D. ______________________

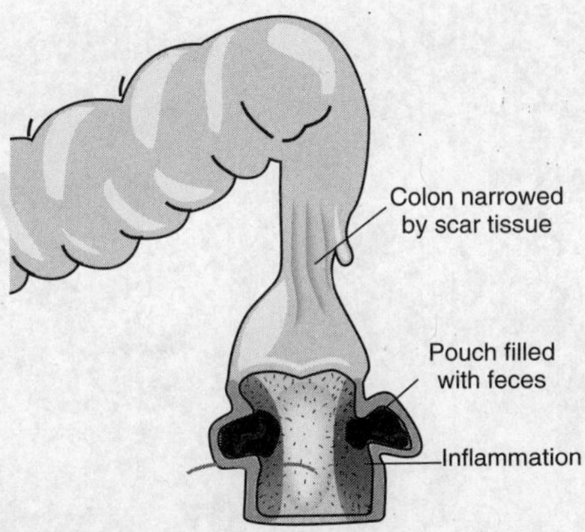

E. ______________________

Copyright © 2027 by Elsevier, Inc. All rights are reserved, including those for text and data mining, AI training, and similar technologies.

61. Outline the **pathophysiology** and **complications** of intestinal obstruction.

62. Describe the signs and symptoms of intestinal obstruction.

63. Define **peritonitis**.

64. Identify the **causes** of peritonitis.

65. Outline the **pathophysiology** and **complications** of peritonitis.

66. Describe the signs and symptoms of peritonitis.

67. List methods/tools used to diagnose peritonitis.

68. Identify the treatment of peritonitis.

CONSOLIDATION

69. Identify the classification of the following medications, and state at least one condition for which each would be prescribed:

   i. prednisone:

   ii. dimenhydrinate:

   iii. clarithromycin:

   iv. ranitidine:

   v. loperamide:

   vi. psyllium:

   vii. sucralfate:

Copyright © 2027 by Elsevier, Inc. All rights are reserved, including those for text and data mining, AI training, and similar technologies.

18 Urinary System Disorders

1. Match the following terms with the organs/structures of the urinary system depicted in the diagram.

   Adrenal gland, Aorta, Hilum, Interior vena cava, Kidney (left), Pelvis, Penis, Prostate gland, Rectum, Renal artery, Renal vein, Ribs, Trigone, Ureter, Ureteral opening, Urethra, Urinary bladder

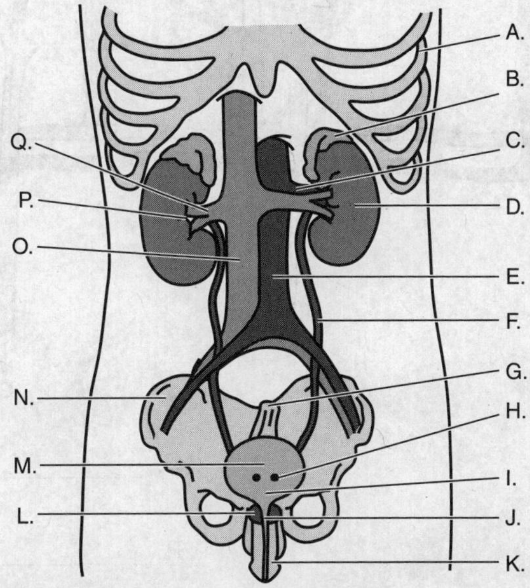

A. ____________________

B. ____________________

C. ____________________

D. ____________________

E. ____________________

F. ____________________

G. ____________________

H. ____________________

I. ____________________

J. ____________________

K. ____________________

L. ____________________

M. ____________________

N. ____________________

O. ____________________

P. ____________________

Q. ____________________

Copyright © 2027 by Elsevier, Inc. All rights are reserved,
including those for text and data mining, AI training, and similar technologies.

2. Match the following terms with the structures of a complete nephron depicted in the diagram.

Afferent arteriole, Arcuate artery, Arcuate vein, Collecting duct, Distal convoluted tubules, Efferent arteriole, Glomerular capillaries, Loop of Henle, Peritubular capillaries, Proximal convoluted tubule, Urine flow

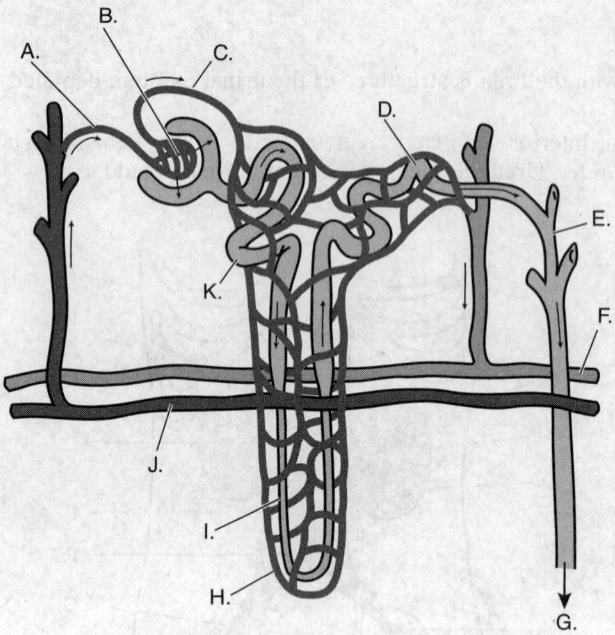

A. ____________________

B. ____________________

C. ____________________

D. ____________________

E. ____________________

F. ____________________

G. ____________________

H. ____________________

I. ____________________

J. ____________________

K. ____________________

3. Urine normally is clear and straw-colored with a mild odor. What are the possible implications of the following?

i. cloudy urine:

ii. dark-colored urine:

iii. urine with an unpleasant or unusual odor:

Copyright © 2027 by Elsevier, Inc. All rights are reserved, including those for text and data mining, AI training, and similar technologies.

4. Name abnormal constituents that may be present in urine.

5. Explain the significance of diuretics and give examples of commonly used diuretics.

6. Explain the difference between **hemodialysis** and **peritoneal dialysis**.

7. Identify **potential complications of hemodialysis**.

8. Explain why individuals receiving hemodialysis are at an **increased risk** of developing HIV and hepatitis B and C.

9. Explain why individuals who require dialysis are usually required to take **prophylactic antibiotics** before dental surgery or other invasive procedures.

10. Identify factors that **predispose** an individual to the development of a **urinary tract infection**. Explain why females are more prone to urinary tract infections than are men.

11. Distinguish between the **manifestations** of **cystitis** and **pyelonephritis**.

12. Describe the **pathophysiology** of **glomerulonephritis**.

13. Outline the signs and symptoms of glomerulonephritis.

14. Identify tests used to **diagnose** glomerulonephritis.

15. Name the possible treatments for glomerulonephritis.

16. Describe the **pathophysiology** of **nephrotic syndrome**.

17. Identify the **most significant sign** of nephrotic syndrome, and outline the potential consequences.

18. List the **medications** used in the treatment of nephrotic syndrome.

19. Identify **causative factors** in the development of **renal calculi**.

Copyright © 2027 by Elsevier, Inc. All rights are reserved,
including those for text and data mining, AI training, and similar technologies.

20. Individuals with renal calculi are routinely instructed to strain their urine. Explain the rationale for this procedure.

21. Identify the characteristic signs and symptoms of renal calculi.

22. Define **hydronephrosis**.

23. Identify **causes** of hydronephrosis.

24. What is a major predisposing factor for the development of malignant tumors in the urinary system?

25. Define **nephrosclerosis**.

26. List the **causes** of nephrosclerosis.

27. Name and briefly describe some congenital disorders of the urinary system.

RENAL FAILURE

28. Identify **causes** of **acute renal failure**.

29. Outline the **treatment** of acute renal failure.

30. Identify **causes** of **chronic renal failure**.

31. Distinguish between **renal insufficiency** and **end-stage renal failure**.

32. Describe the **manifestations** of end-stage renal failure under the following headings:

    i. fluid and electrolyte balance:

    ii. cardiovascular system:

    iii. central nervous system:

    iv. musculoskeletal system:

Copyright © 2027 by Elsevier, Inc. All rights are reserved, including those for text and data mining, AI training, and similar technologies.

v. endocrine system:

vi. skin and mucosa:

33. Explain why each of the following manifestations occurs in end-stage renal failure:

i. metabolic acidosis:

ii. hyperkalemia:

iii. hypocalcemia:

iv. increased blood urea nitrogen (BUN) and serum creatinine:

v. anemia:

vi. delayed clotting:

vii. edema:

viii. increased blood pressure:

ix. cardiac dysrhythmias:

x. congestive heart failure:

xi. pulmonary edema:

xii. lethargy, confusion:

xiii. muscle weakness:

xiv. bone pain:

xv. amenorrhea:

xvi. severe pruritus:

xvii. ammonia odor on breath:

xviii. hypoplasia of tooth enamel:

Copyright © 2027 by Elsevier, Inc. All rights are reserved,
including those for text and data mining, AI training, and similar technologies.

34. Explain why individuals with renal failure have an increased chance of having an exaggerated or prolonged response to many medications.

35. Complete the following crossword puzzle:

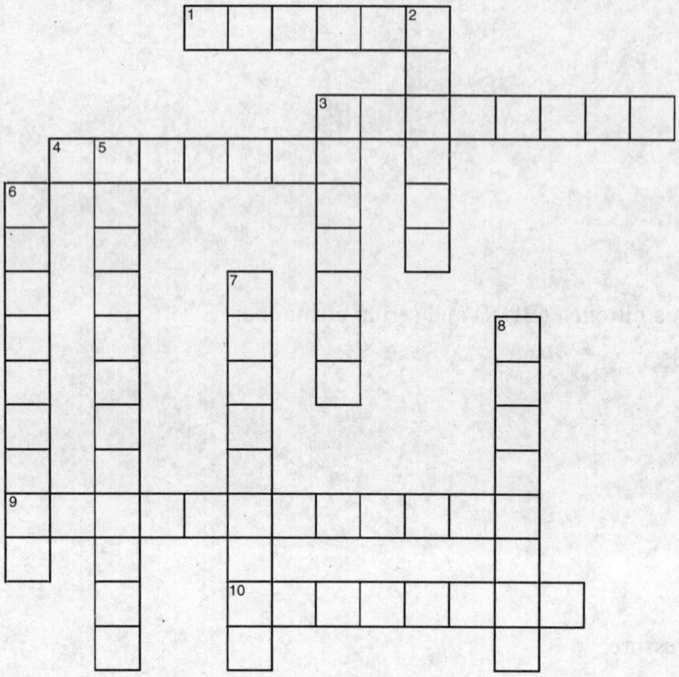

ACROSS

1. presence of pus in the urine
3. medication that promotes urination
4. sudden, extreme urge to void
9. inability to control urination
10. scanty urine output

DOWN

2. no urine output
3. painful urination
5. kidney stones
6. blood in the urine
7. Inability to empty bladder
8. presence of nitrogenous wastes in blood

Copyright © 2027 by Elsevier, Inc. All rights are reserved, including those for text and data mining, AI training, and similar technologies.

19 Reproductive System Disorders

1. Identify causes of **infertility** for both males and females.

MALES

2. Match the following terms with the organs/structures of the male reproductive system depicted in the diagram.

Ampulla, Bulbourethral gland, Ductus deferens, Ejaculatory duct, Epididymis, Glans penis, Membranous urethra, Parietal peritoneal membrane, Penis, Prepuce (foreskin), Prostate gland, Prostatic urethra, Rectum, Scrotum, Seminal vesicle, Seminiferous tubules, Spongy urethra, Surface of urinary bladder, Testis, Ureter, Urethra, Urinary bladder opened

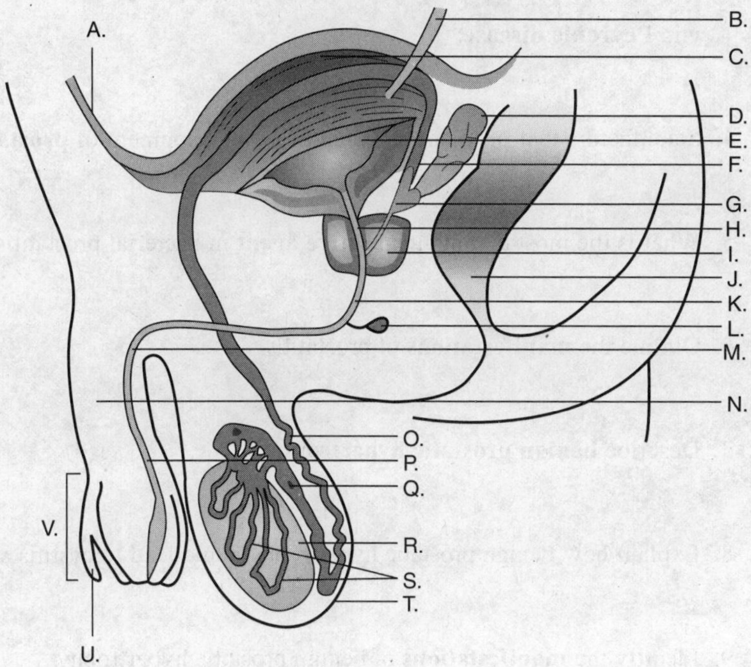

A. ______________________

B. ______________________

C. ______________________

D. ______________________

E. ______________________

F. ______________________

G. ______________________

H. ______________________

I. ______________________

J. ______________________

K. ______________________

L. ______________________

M. ______________________

N. ______________________

O. ______________________

P. ______________________

Q. ______________________

R. ______________________

S. ______________________

T. ______________________

U. ______________________

V. ______________________

Copyright © 2027 by Elsevier, Inc. All rights are reserved, including those for text and data mining, AI training, and similar technologies.

3. Define the following terms/conditions:

   i. **hypospadias**:

   ii. **epispadias**:

   iii. **cryptorchidism**:

   iv. **hydrocele**:

   v. **spermatocele**:

   vi. **varicocele**:

   vii. **Peyronie disease**:

4. State factors that **predispose** a man to the development of **prostatitis**.

5. What is the most common **causative agent** in bacterial prostatitis?

6. Outline the **manifestations** of prostatitis.

7. Describe **benign prostatic hypertrophy**.

8. Explain how benign prostatic hypertrophy could lead to cystitis and kidney damage.

9. Identify the **manifestations** of benign prostatic hypertrophy.

10. What are the **risk factors** associated with the development of **prostatic cancer**?

11. What are the **warning or early signs** of **prostatic cancer**?

12. Prostatic cancer often metastasizes. Identify common **sites of metastases**.

13. What **screening tools** are useful in the early detection of prostatic cancer?

Copyright © 2027 by Elsevier, Inc. All rights are reserved, including those for text and data mining, AI training, and similar technologies.

14. Why are testosterone blocking agents sometimes useful in the treatment of prostatic cancer?

15. List known **risk factors** for **testicular cancer**.

16. Describe the **manifestations** of testicular cancer.

17. Outline **therapeutic interventions** used in the treatment of testicular cancer.

FEMALE

18. Match the following terms with the organs/structures of the female reproductive system depicted in the diagram.

Anus, Cervix, Clitoris, Coccyx, Fallopian tube, Fimbriae, Labium majus, Labium minus, Ovary, Peritoneal membrane, Posterior fornix, Rectum, Symphysis pubis, Urethra, Urinary bladder, Uterus, Vagina, Vaginal orifice

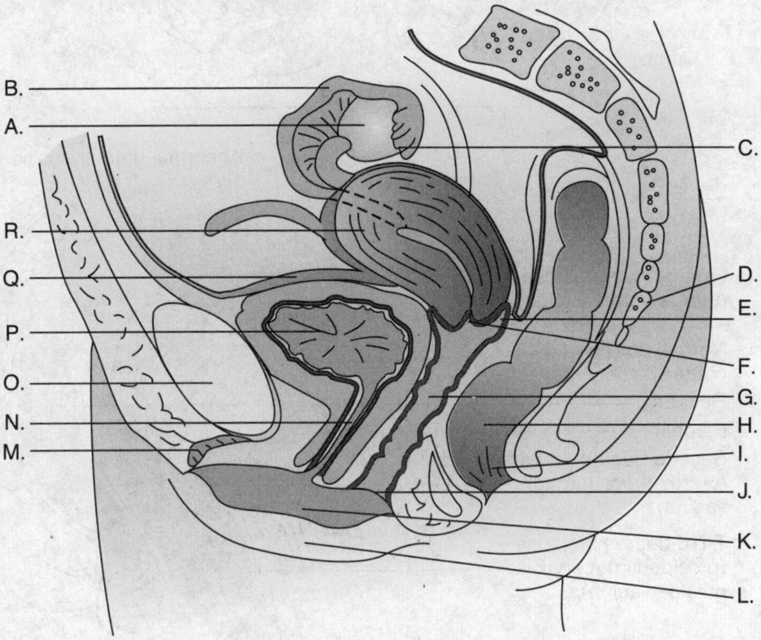

A. ____________________

B. ____________________

C. ____________________

D. ____________________

E. ____________________

F. ____________________

G. ____________________

H. ____________________

I. ____________________

J. ____________________

K. ____________________

L. ____________________

M. ____________________

N. ____________________

O. ____________________

P. ____________________

Q. ____________________

R. ____________________

Copyright © 2027 by Elsevier, Inc. All rights are reserved, including those for text and data mining, AI training, and similar technologies.

19. Define the following terms:

i. **dysmenorrhea**:

ii. **amenorrhea**:

iii. **dyspareunia**:

20. Match the following terms with the diagrams depicting structural abnormalities of the uterus.

Anteflexion, Cystocele, Rectocele, Retrocession, Retroflexion-flexion posteriorly, Retroversion, Uterine prolapse

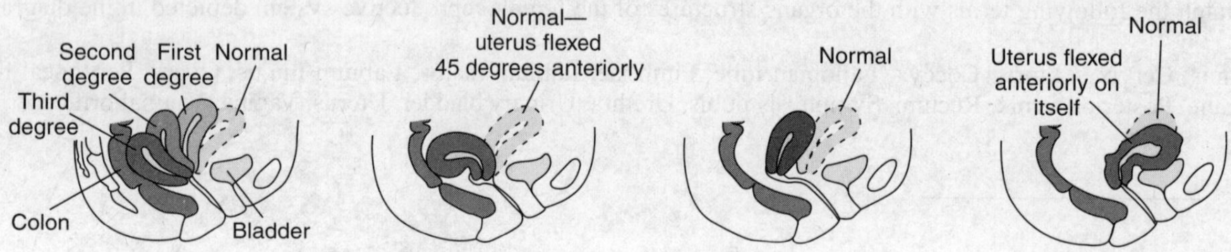

A. ______________ B. ______________ C. ______________ D. ______________

Abnormal uterine positions

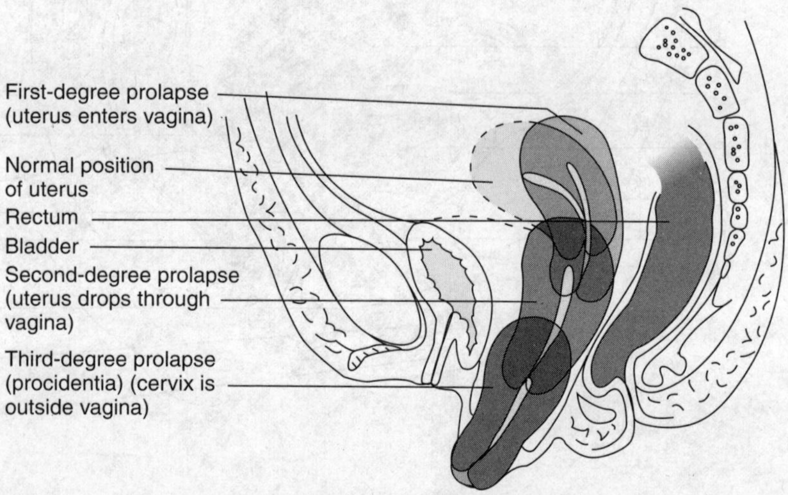

E. ______________

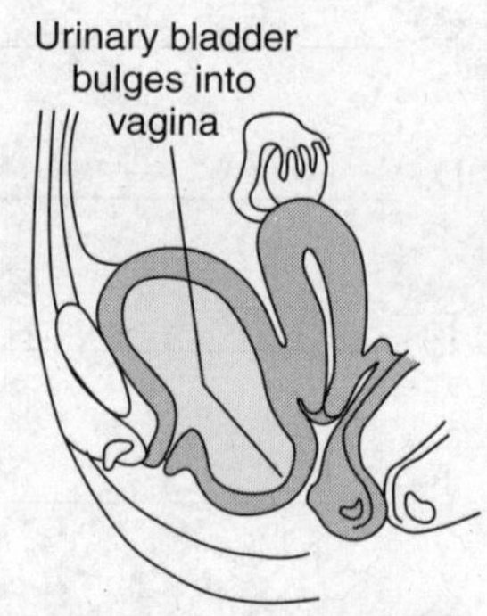

G. ______________

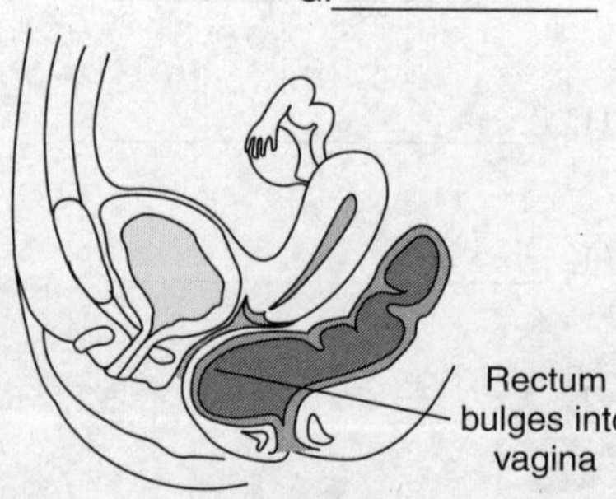

F. ______________

21. Briefly list six steps in the menstrual cycle.

Copyright © 2027 by Elsevier, Inc. All rights are reserved,
including those for text and data mining, AI training, and similar technologies.

ENDOMETRIOSIS

22. Define **endometriosis**.

23. Describe the **pathophysiology** of endometriosis.

24. Identify the **primary manifestation** with endometriosis.

25. Outline the **treatment** for endometriosis.

VAGINAL CANDIDIASIS

26. Identify **predisposing factors** for the development of **vaginal candidiasis**. Note that these are exactly the same factors that predispose an individual to oral candidiasis.

27. Outline the **manifestations** of vaginal candidiasis.

PELVIC INFLAMMATORY DISEASE

28. Define **pelvic inflammatory disease (PID)**.

29. Identify **predisposing factors** for the development of PID.

30. Describe the **pathophysiology** of PID.

31. Outline the **manifestations** of PID.

32. Identify the potential complications of untreated PID.

33. What is the **treatment** for PID?

BREAST CANCER

34. Identify **risk factors** for breast cancer.

35. Outline the **development** of breast cancer, including the **metastatic pattern**.

Copyright © 2027 by Elsevier, Inc. All rights are reserved, including those for text and data mining, AI training, and similar technologies.

36. Identify the **manifestations** of breast cancer.

37. Outline the **therapeutic interventions** used in the treatment of breast cancer.

38. Discuss measures that can be used to detect **early signs** of breast cancer.

CERVICAL CANCER

39. Explain why the number of deaths from cervical cancer has declined. Why has the incidence of new cases not decreased?

40. Identify individuals who are considered at **high risk** for developing cervical cancer.

41. Describe the **progression** of undiagnosed or untreated cervical cancer.

42. List the **signs and symptoms** of cervical cancer.

43. Outline the **treatment** for cervical cancer.

ENDOMETRIAL CANCER

44. Identify individuals who are considered at **high risk** for developing endometrial cancer.

45. Describe the **progression** of undiagnosed or untreated endometrial cancer.

46. List the **manifestations** of endometrial cancer.

47. Outline the **treatment** of endometrial cancer.

Copyright © 2027 by Elsevier, Inc. All rights are reserved, including those for text and data mining, AI training, and similar technologies.

SEXUALLY TRANSMITTED DISEASES

48. Complete the following chart comparing and contrasting different sexually transmitted diseases:

Infection	Causative Agent	Manifestations	Complications	Treatment
Chlamydia				
Gonorrhea				
Syphilis				
Genital herpes				
Genital warts				
Trichomoniasis				

Copyright © 2027 by Elsevier, Inc. All rights are reserved,
including those for text and data mining, AI training, and similar technologies.

20 Neoplasms and Cancer

1. Define the following terms:

   i. neoplasm:

   ii. benign:

   iii. malignant:

   iv. carcinoma:

   v. sarcoma:

   vi. anaplasia:

2. Name three specific pathophysiological changes that occur in the formation of malignant tumors.

3. Identify the correct nomenclature for both benign and malignant tumors in the following tissues/organs:

	Benign Tumor	Malignant Tumor
Pancreas		
Fat		
Bone		
Liver		
Cartilage		
Skin		

Copyright © 2027 by Elsevier, Inc. All rights are reserved, including those for text and data mining, AI training, and similar technologies.

4. Compare and contrast benign and malignant tumors using the following chart:

	Benign Tumors	Malignant Tumors
Cells		
Growth		
Spread		
Systemic effects		
General prognosis		

5. Describe how the study of telomeres and the enzyme telomerase is relevant to both the process of cellular aging and the development of cancer.

6. A tumor is a space-occupying mass that produces predictable local effects as it enlarges. Describe the **consequences** that could result from the following effects:

i. compression of blood vessels:

ii. compression or obstruction of a tube or duct:

iii. compression of nerves:

iv. erosion of blood vessels and other structures:

v. invasion and replacement of normal tissue:

Copyright © 2027 by Elsevier, Inc. All rights are reserved,
including those for text and data mining, AI training, and similar technologies.

7. Malignant tumors also have **generalized systemic effects**. Outline the factors that contribute to the development of the following systemic manifestations:

   i. weight loss and cachexia:

   ii. anemia:

   iii. systemic infections:

   iv. bleeding:

8. Define and describe **paraneoplastic syndrome**.

9. Explain how the following diagnostic tools can assist in the detection and diagnosis of cancer:

   i. blood tests:

   ii. tumor markers:

   iii. x-ray, ultrasound, magnetic resonance imaging, and computed tomography scan:

   iv. biopsy and histological and cytological examinations:

10. Describe how malignant cells **spread** from the original tumor to distant sites in the body. What is this called?

11. Distinguish between the **grading** and **staging** of neoplasms.

12. Differentiate between an **initiating factor** and a **promoter** in relation to carcinogenesis.

13. Identify eight **risk factors** for developing cancer and include at least one example of each.

14. Explain why individuals who have incompetent immune systems are at a higher risk of developing malignancies.

15. Identify the four conventional treatment measures employed in the treatment of cancer. Why are they often used in combination rather than singly?

Copyright © 2027 by Elsevier, Inc. All rights are reserved, including those for text and data mining, AI training, and similar technologies.

16. Treatment for cancer may be **curative**, **palliative**, or **prophylactic**. Explain the circumstances when each of these treatments may be used.

17. Explain how **radiotherapy** is effective in treating some types of cancer.

18. Identify the mechanisms of action of **antineoplastic medications**.

19. Identify **adverse effects** that commonly occur during both radiotherapy and chemotherapy, and explain why they happen.

20. What are three factors that contribute to malnutrition in patients with advanced cancer?

21. What is a **biologic response modifier**? How are these agents useful in the treatment of some types of cancer?

22. Explain the three potential goals of gene therapy in the treatment of cancer.

23. Identify **other types of drugs** that may be used in the treatment of cancer, including the rationale for each.

24. What is the most common form of **skin cancer**?

Copyright © 2027 by Elsevier, Inc. All rights are reserved, including those for text and data mining, AI training, and similar technologies.

25. Complete the following crossword puzzle:

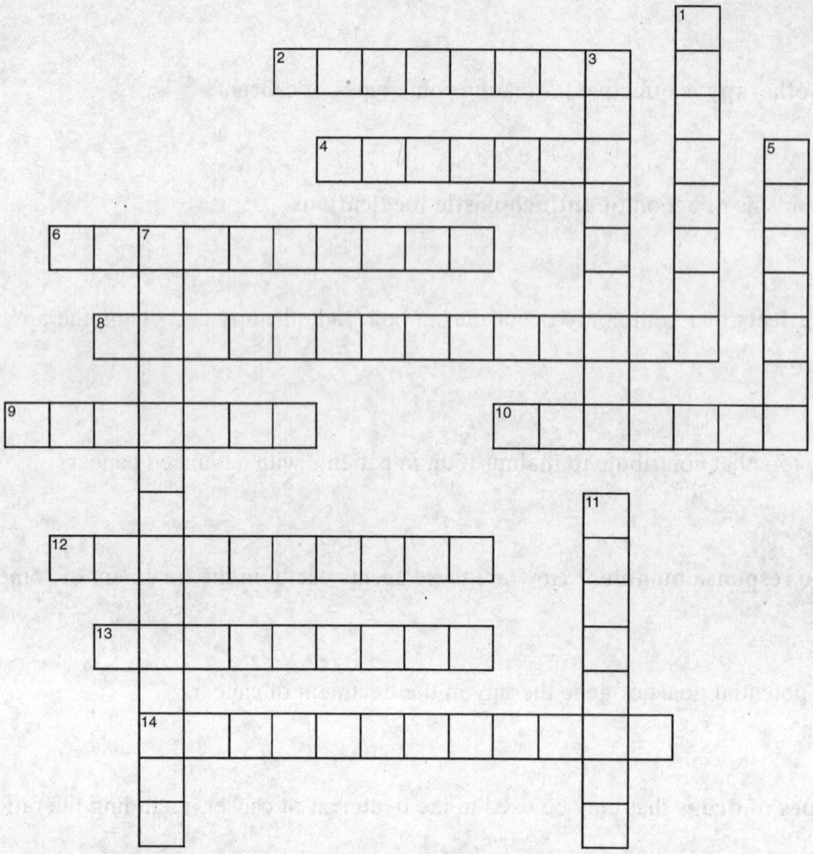

ACROSS

2. severe tissue wasting
4. malignant tumor arising from connective tissue
6. spread of cancer to a distant site
8. transformation of normal cells into cancer cells
9. confined to the site of origin (hyphenated)
10. degree of differentiation of malignant cells
12. cancer-causing agent
13. malignant tumor arising in epithelial tissue
14. invasion

DOWN

1. agents capable of causing alterations in DNA
3. failure of cells to develop specialized features
5. spread of cancer via body secretions
7. conversion of normal cells to cancerous cells
11. the study of cancer

Copyright © 2027 by Elsevier, Inc. All rights reserved, including those for text and data mining, AI training, and similar technologies.

21 Congenital and Genetic Disorders

1. Define **congenital anomalies**.

2. Outline the etiology of **chromosomal disorders**.

3. Define **teratogenic agents**.

4. Differentiate between an **inherited disorder** and a **chromosomal disorder**.

5. Name and briefly describe single-gene disorders.

6. Define each of the following terms:

   i. **monosomy**:

   ii. **trisomy**:

7. Explain what is meant by a **"multifactorial disorder."** Identify several examples.

8. Explain how maternal substance abuse might cause developmental disorders, and identify the most critical time of embryonic development for such effects.

9. Explain how a congenital disorder might occur as a result of factors during labor and delivery.

10. What is a significant **risk factor** for chromosomal disorders?

11. Explain the difference between the **carrier** of an infectious disease such as hepatitis B and the carrier of a genetic disorder.

12. In what type or types of inherited disorders is there a **carrier** state?

Copyright © 2027 by Elsevier, Inc. All rights are reserved,
including those for text and data mining, AI training, and similar technologies.

13. What is the genotype of a carrier: heterozygous or homozygous? Does a carrier of a genetic disorder usually become symptomatic?

14. Let "H" represent an **autosomal dominant disorder**. Complete the following Punnett square, and then answer the accompanying questions:

		Father	
		H	h
Mother	h		
	h		

i. Which parent is affected by this disorder: the father or mother?

ii. What is the probability that this couple will produce a child with the disorder?

iii. What is the probability that this couple will produce a child who is a carrier of the disease? Explain.

15. Let "H" represent an **autosomal dominant disorder**. Complete the following Punnett square, and then answer the accompanying questions:

		Father	
		H	h
Mother	H		
	h		

i. Which parent is affected by this disorder?

ii. What is the probability that this couple will produce a child with the disease?

16. Let "t" represent an **autosomal recessive disorder**. Complete the following Punnett square, and then answer the accompanying questions:

		Father	
		T	T
Mother	T		
	t		

Copyright © 2027 by Elsevier, Inc. All rights are reserved, including those for text and data mining, AI training, and similar technologies.

i. Which parent is:

a) affected by this disorder?

b) a carrier of this disorder?

c) asymptomatic in relation to this disorder?

ii. What is the probability that this couple will produce a child:

a) with the disorder?

b) who is a carrier of the disorder?

c) who is phenotypically normal?

d) who is not a carrier?

17. Let "t" represent an **autosomal recessive disorder**. Complete the following Punnett square, and then answer the accompanying questions:

		Father	
		T	t
Mother	T		
	t		

i. Which parent is:

a) affected by this disorder?

b) a carrier of this disorder?

c) asymptomatic in relation to this disorder?

ii. What is the probability that this couple will produce a child:

a) with the disorder?

b) who is a carrier of the disorder?

c) who is phenotypically normal?

d) who is not a carrier?

Copyright © 2027 by Elsevier, Inc. All rights are reserved,
including those for text and data mining, AI training, and similar technologies.

18. Let "t" represent an **autosomal recessive disorder**. Complete the following Punnett square, and then answer the accompanying questions:

Father

		t	t
Mother	T		
	t		

i. Which parent is:

a) affected by this disorder?

b) a carrier of this disorder?

c) asymptomatic in relation to this disorder?

ii. What is the probability that this couple will produce a child:

a) with the disorder?

b) who is a carrier of the disorder?

c) who is phenotypically normal?

d) who is not a carrier?

19. A newborn is diagnosed with phenylketonuria (PKU), an autosomal recessive disorder. Neither of his parents has this disease.

i. What is the baby's genotype?

ii. Which parent is a carrier of PKU?

iii. If this couple has a second child, what is the probability that they will also have phenylketonuria?

iv. What is the probability that any of the baby's siblings will be carriers of phenylketonuria?

Copyright © 2027 by Elsevier, Inc. All rights are reserved, including those for text and data mining, AI training, and similar technologies.

20. Let "t" represent an **autosomal recessive disorder.** Complete the following Punnett square, and then answer the accompanying questions:

Father

Mother	t	t
t		
t		

i. Which parent is:

a) affected by this disorder?

b) a carrier of this disorder?

c) asymptomatic in relation to this disorder?

ii. What is the probability that this couple will produce a child:

a) with the disorder?

b) who is a carrier of the disorder?

c) who is phenotypically normal?

d) who is not a carrier?

21. **Sex-linked disorders** are often referred to as "X-linked" because the abnormal gene is usually carried on the X chromosome. Let "H" represent the normal gene and "h" the abnormal one. Complete the following Punnett squares, and then answer the accompanying questions:

Square A

	X^H	Y
X^H		
X^h		

Referring to Square A:

i. Which parent is:

a) affected by this disorder?

b) a carrier of this disorder?

ii. What is the probability that this couple will produce a child with the disorder?

Copyright © 2027 by Elsevier, Inc. All rights are reserved,
including those for text and data mining, AI training, and similar technologies.

iii. What would be the sex of that child?

iv. What is the probability that this couple will produce a child who is a carrier of this disorder? What would be the sex of that child?

v. What is the probability of producing a genotypically and phenotypically normal:

a) son?

b) daughter?

Square B

	X^h	Y
X^h		
X^H		

Referring to Square B:

i. Which parent is:

a) affected by this disorder?

b) a carrier of this disorder?

c) genotypically and phenotypically normal?

ii. What is the probability that this couple's:

a) daughters will be carriers of this disorder?

b) daughters will be affected by this disorder?

c) sons will be carriers of this disorder?

d) sons will be affected by this disorder?

22. How could a female individual have a sex-linked disorder? Draw a Punnett square to illustrate this scenario.

23. A boy is diagnosed with Duchenne muscular dystrophy, a sex-linked disorder. Neither of his parents has this disease.

i. What is the child's genotype?

ii. Which parent is a carrier?

Copyright © 2027 by Elsevier, Inc. All rights reserved, including those for text and data mining, AI training, and similar technologies.

iii. If this couple has a second child, what is the probability that they will also have cystic fibrosis?

iv. If the child does have a sibling with muscular dystrophy, will it be a brother or sister? Explain.

v. What is the probability that any of the child's siblings will be carriers of cystic fibrosis? Will the carriers be male or female? Explain.

24. Select the appropriate classification for each of these genetic disorders.
Classifications: Chromosomal, Autosomal dominant, Autosomal recessive, X-linked dominant, X-linked recessive, multifactorial

i. fragile X syndrome:

ii. cystic fibrosis:

iii. adult polycystic kidney disease:

iv. familial hypercholesterolemia:

v. Duchenne muscular dystrophy:

vi. sickle cell anemia:

vii. hemophilia A:

viii. Klinefelter syndrome:

ix. phenylketonuria:

x. Huntington disease:

xi. Tay-Sachs disease:

xii. schizophrenia:

xiii. cleft lip and palate:

xiv. Turner syndrome:

Copyright © 2027 by Elsevier, Inc. All rights are reserved,
including those for text and data mining, AI training, and similar technologies.

25. What type of disorder is **Down syndrome**? How can it be diagnosed prenatally? What is the karyotype of an individual with Down syndrome?

26. Outline the abnormalities or problems associated with Down syndrome.

27. Describe the characteristic appearance of an individual with Down syndrome.

28. Describe Turner Syndrome.

29. Describe Klinefelter Syndrome.

Copyright © 2027 by Elsevier, Inc. All rights are reserved, including those for text and data mining, AI training, and similar technologies.

22 Complications of Pregnancy

1. Identify the time periods for the embryonic stage, **fetal** stage, and **organogenesis** in pregnancy.

2. Discuss the risk to a developing fetus if the mother smokes during the pregnancy.

3. What is the hormone used as the basis for laboratory diagnosis of pregnancy, and how accurate is the test in each of the trimesters?

4. Match the following definitions with the correct terms:

a) milk production	i. **gestation**
b) pregnancy	ii. gravidity
c) inflammation of uterine lining	iii. **parity**
d) number of pregnancies	iv. lactation
e) number of viable pregnancies	v. endometritis

5. Briefly describe the following complications of pregnancy:

   i. ectopic pregnancy:

   ii. preeclampsia and eclampsia:

   iii. gestational diabetes mellitus:

   iv. placenta previa:

   v. abruption placentae:

   vi. thromboembolism:

   vii. disseminated intravascular coagulation:

Copyright © 2027 by Elsevier, Inc. All rights are reserved,
including those for text and data mining, AI training, and similar technologies.

viii. Rh incompatibility:

ix. infections:

x. adolescent pregnancy:

6. Explain why **Rh incompatibility** occurs. Describe the manifestations and complications of Rh incompatibility.

7. Define **RhoGAM** and explain how it prevents Rh incompatibility complications in subsequent pregnancies.

8. Name and explain risks that can occur during adolescent pregnancies.

Copyright © 2027 by Elsevier, Inc. All rights are reserved,
including those for text and data mining, AI training, and similar technologies.

23 Complications of Adolescence

1. Define the period of adolescence.

2. Using a body mass index (BMI) chart, calculate the BMI for the individuals listed below. In addition, determine whether the BMI of the individual is normal (N), overweight (Ov), or obese (Ob).

Height	Pounds (lb)	BMI	N, Ov, Ob
4'7"	130		
4'7"	100		
4'11"	100		
5'2"	140		
5'7"	180		
5'7"	210		

3. Name the pathophysiological problems associated with obesity in children and teens.

4. Name the three factors that are common in definitions for **"metabolic syndrome."**

5. Match the following definitions with the correct terms:

a) condition characterized by alternating "binge and purge" behavior

b) extreme weight loss caused by self-starvation

c) demineralization of bone

d) bone infection

i. osteoporosis

ii. osteomyelitis

iii. anorexia nervosa

iv. bulimia nervosa

Copyright © 2027 by Elsevier, Inc. All rights are reserved,
including those for text and data mining, AI training, and similar technologies.

6. Match terms with abnormal curvature of spine depicted in the diagrams.

Kyphosis, Lordosis, Scoliosis

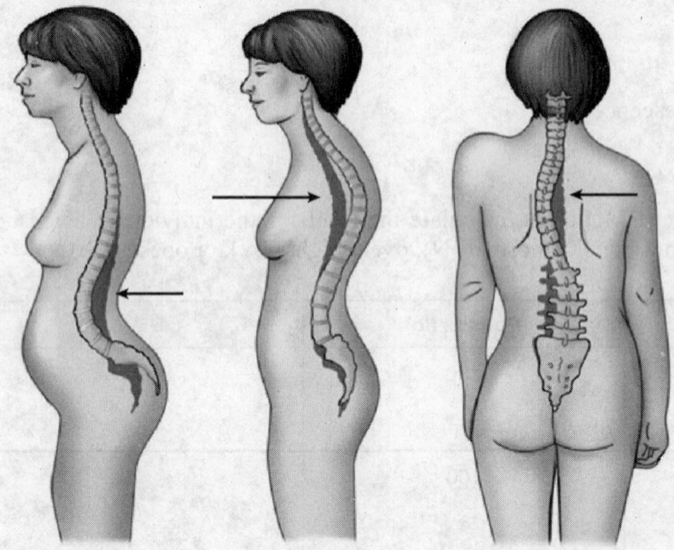

A.____________ B.____________ C.____________

From Patton KT, et al: *The human body in health and disease,* ed. 8, St. Louis, 2024, Elsevier.

7. Identify **risk factors** for the development of **osteomyelitis**.

8. Outline the **pathophysiology** of osteomyelitis.

9. Juvenile rheumatoid arthritis (JRA), an autoimmune disease, is somewhat similar in pathology to adult rheumatoid arthritis. What are the distinctive characteristics of JRA?

10. Describe treatments for JRA.

11. Distinguish between **anorexia nervosa** and **bulimia nervosa**.

12. What two organisms are most often associated with acne vulgaris?

13. What is the causative agent of **mononucleosis**?

14. List the **manifestations and potential complications** of mononucleosis.

15. Which chromosomal disorder in females is caused by a lack of an X chromosome, and how does this affect sexual development?

16. What is the definition of *dysmenorrhea*?

Copyright © 2027 by Elsevier, Inc. All rights reserved, including those for text and data mining, AI training, and similar technologies.

24 Complications of Aging

1. Identify three theories of aging discussed in the text and briefly explain how each contributes to the aging process.

2. Describe the **effects of aging** on the following body systems:

   i. Endocrine:

   ii. Reproductive, both female and male:

   iii. Skin and mucosa:

   iv. Cardiovascular:

   v. Musculoskeletal:

   vi. Respiratory:

   vii. Nervous:

   viii. Gastrointestinal:

   ix. Urinary:

3. Explain physiologically why elderly people are at a higher risk for infections and cancer than are younger individuals.

Copyright © 2027 by Elsevier, Inc. All rights are reserved,
including those for text and data mining, AI training, and similar technologies.

4. Match the following definitions with the correct terms:

a) inability to control urination	i. atherosclerosis
b) farsightedness	ii. cataract
c) predetermined cell death	iii. apoptosis
d) excessive urination at night	iv. glaucoma
e) opacity of the ocular lens	v. incontinence
f) deposition of fat in arterial walls	vi. nocturia
g) dry mouth	vii. presbyopia
h) increased intraocular pressure	viii. xerostomia

Copyright © 2027 by Elsevier, Inc. All rights reserved, including those for text and data mining, AI training, and similar technologies.

25 Immobility and Associated Problems

1. Summarize the **effects of immobility** throughout the body systems.

2. Match the following definitions with the correct terms:

a) stationary blood clot	i. atelectasis
b) collapse of lung tissue	ii. contracture
c) sudden drop in blood pressure when change in position occurs	iii. decubitus ulcer
d) break away thrombus	iv. embolus
e) pressure sore or bedsore	v. hemiplegia
f) paralysis below the waist	vi. orthostatic hypotension
g) joint deformity caused by excessive scarring	vii. paraplegia
h) paralysis of one side of the body	viii. thrombus
i) loss of bone mass	ix. flaccidity
j) loss of muscle tone	x. osteoporosis

3. Name two classes of drugs that may lead to slowed, shallow respiration, especially in immobilized persons.

4. Identify the major digestive system complication caused by immobility and treatments.

5. Identify urinary system complications caused by immobility.

Copyright © 2027 by Elsevier, Inc. All rights are reserved,
including those for text and data mining, AI training, and similar technologies.

26 Stress and Associated Problems

1. Define the term **stressor** and provide two examples.

2. Each individual may perceive stress differently. Identify two factors that may impair an individual's ability to respond effectively to a stressor.

3. Identify the **hormones** that are secreted during the stress response, including the source and effects of each.

4. Describe three effects of the **sympathetic nervous system** activation during the stress response.

5. Explain how prolonged stress, such as that from divorce or professional difficulties, can contribute to specific health problems

6. Name three strategies/support systems that may play a role in minimizing the risk of the development of stress-related pathologies.

7. Define **technostress**.

8. Describe the three stages of the general adaptation syndrome and explain how each stage affects the body's response to stress.

Copyright © 2027 by Elsevier, Inc. All rights are reserved, including those for text and data mining, AI training, and similar technologies.

27 Substance Abuse and Associated Problems

1. What is the basic difference between the terms **physiological dependence**, **psychological dependence**, and **addiction**?

2. According to present theories, what are the five causes of substance abuse?

3. Describe the three stages of liver damage that may be caused by excessive alcohol intake (Laënnec cirrhosis).

4. Name medications used to treat heroin addiction and alcohol addiction.

5. Identify the primary antidote currently available to treat opioid overdoses.

6. Match each of the following street drug names with the drug clinical name.

a) Speed	i. methamphetamine
b) Ecstasy	ii. phencyclidine
c) Blow	iii. nicotine
d) Angel dust	iv. amphetamines
e) Ice	v. MDMA
f) Snow	vi. marijuana
g) Special K	vii. cocaine
h) Weed	viii. heroin

Copyright © 2027 by Elsevier, Inc. All rights are reserved,
including those for text and data mining, AI training, and similar technologies.

28 Environmental Hazards and Associated Problems

1. Identify three mechanisms by which chemicals can damage cells in the body.

2. Identify four toxic effects of lead exposure on the human body, including the specific tissues or systems affected.

3. What are the two classifications of chemical **inhalants**? Give an example of each.

4. What is **hyperthermia**? List three syndromes associated with **hyperthermia**.

5. Describe some of the differences between local and systemic **hypothermia**.

6. What types of body cells does **radiation** primarily affect?

7. List three ways in which a bite or sting may cause disease.

8. Describe two food- or water-borne pathogens and their associated health effects.

9. Explain how excessive noise exposure can lead to hearing loss and other physiological effects.

Copyright © 2027 by Elsevier, Inc. All rights are reserved, including those for text and data mining, AI training, and similar technologies.

Answer Key

CHAPTER 1: Introduction to Pathophysiology

1. This is basically a three-step process before a new therapy can be approved.
   First stage: "basic science"
   Second stage: determination if therapy is safe for humans (clinical trial with a small number of human subjects)
   Third stage: more clinical trials with double-blind studies
   See detailed explanation in the chapter.
2. An approved therapy may show additional benefits to treat a different disease. A recent example for "off-label" use is the use of hydroxychloroquine, a drug approved for the treatment and prevention of malaria and now also used by some physicians in the fight against SARS-CoV-2.
3. AI in health care is an addition to the information management for both the physician and the patient. It can be used to diagnose disease, enhance treatment, and design new drugs more efficiently.
4. *acute disease:* a short-term illness that develops quickly; *chronic disease:* a milder condition that develops gradually but persists for a long time and usually causes more permanent tissue damage.
5. *epidemic:* higher than expected number of cases of an infectious disease within a given area; *pandemic:* higher number of cases in many regions of the globe.
6.
   i. atrophy
   ii. hyperplasia
   iii. hypertrophy
   iv. neoplasia
   v. neoplasia
   vi. atrophy
   vii. atrophy
   viii. metaplasia
   ix. dysplasia
   x. hyperplasia
   xi. metaplasia; dysplasia; neoplasia
   xii. hyperplasia
   xiii. hypertrophy
   xiv. hyperplasia
   xv. atrophy
   xvi. hyperplasia
7. dysplasia; may be the forerunner of neoplasia
8. failure of cells to differentiate or develop specialized features; term applied to grading malignant tumors
9.
   i. ischemia
   ii. physical agents (e.g., excessive temperature, radiation)
   iii. mechanical damage
   iv. chemical toxins or foreign substances
   v. pathogens
   vi. abnormal metabolites
   vii. nutritional deficits
   viii. fluid or electrolyte imbalances
10. answers to crossword puzzle
11.
   a. Atrophy
   b. Normal cells
   c. Hyperplasia
   d. Dysplasia
   e. Hypertrophy
   f. Metaplasia
   g. Neoplasia (malignancy)

Copyright © 2027 by Elsevier, Inc. All rights are reserved, including those for text and data mining, AI training, and similar technologies.

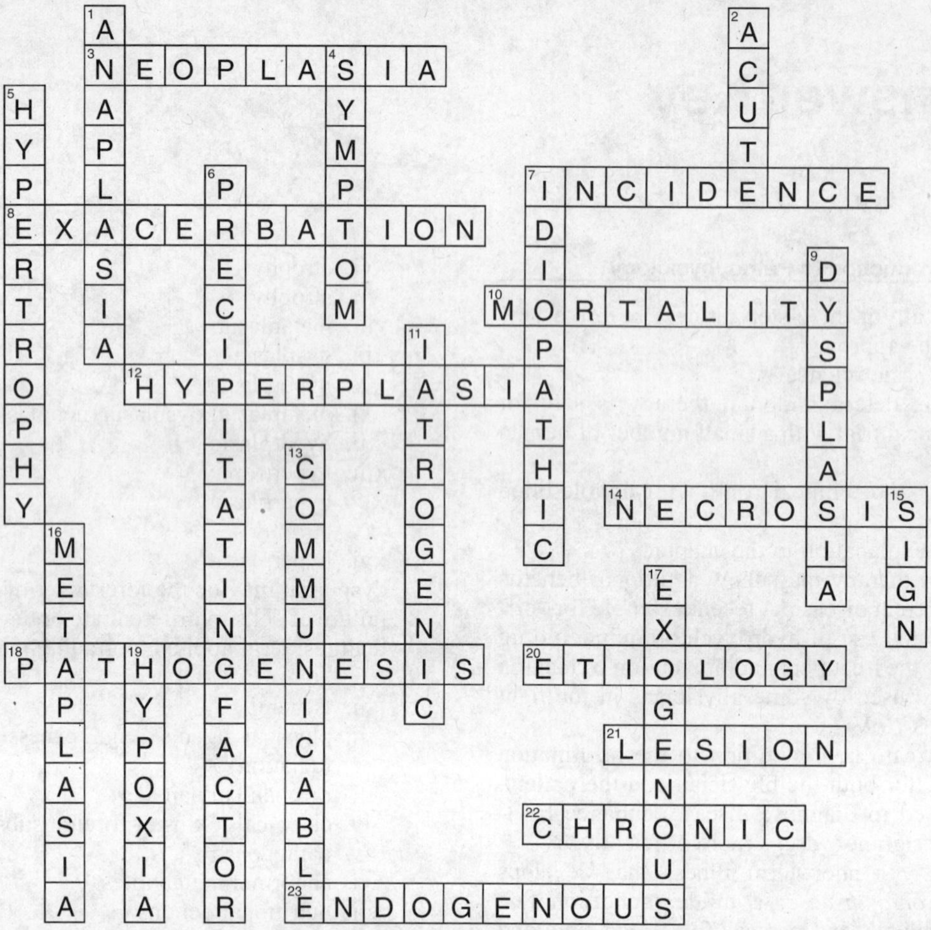

CHAPTER 2: Fluid, Electrolyte, and Acid-Base Imbalances

EDEMA

1. excess fluid in the interstitial compartment
2. (Fig. 2.2)
   i. increased capillary hydrostatic pressure, forcing excessive amounts of fluid out and preventing return of fluid from the interstitial compartment
   ii. loss of plasma proteins, reducing plasma osmotic pressure
   iii. obstruction of lymphatic circulation, restricting the return of excess fluid and protein to the general circulation
   iv. increased capillary permeability—as in inflammation, resulting in fluid and protein movement into the interstitial compartment
3.
   i. obstruction of lymphatic circulation due to removal of lymphatic vessels; increased capillary permeability, and increased capillary hydrostatic pressure immediately following surgery
   ii. loss of plasma proteins due to decreased production of plasma proteins
   iii. increased capillary hydrostatic pressure and increased capillary permeability
   iv. increased capillary hydrostatic pressure caused by/due to increased blood volume; possibly caused by/due to decreased capillary osmotic pressure due to protein-wasting kidney disease
   v. increased capillary hydrostatic pressure caused by/due to the effects of gravity
   vi. increased capillary hydrostatic pressure and increased capillary permeability caused by/due to inflammation
   vii. obstruction of lymphatic circulation or increased capillary hydrostatic pressure if blood vessels are compressed
   viii. increased capillary permeability and loss of plasma proteins
   ix. increased capillary hydrostatic pressure caused by/due to increased water retention
   x. loss of plasma proteins caused by/due to decreased synthesis of plasma proteins
   xi. increased capillary hydrostatic pressure
   xii. increased capillary hydrostatic pressure and increased capillary permeability caused by/due to inflammation
4. (Table 2.3) local swelling; pale, gray or red skin color; pitting edema; slow, bounding pulse with high

Copyright © 2027 by Elsevier, Inc. All rights are reserved, including those for text and data mining, AI training, and similar technologies.

blood pressure; lethargy, possible seizures; pulmonary congestion, cough, rales; weight gain; functional impairment of joints or movement of organs such as the heart and lungs; pain; impairment of arterial circulation; tissue breakdown from pressure, abrasion, and external chemicals; infection of gingival tissue

DEHYDRATION

5. vomiting, diarrhea, excessive sweating, diabetic ketoacidosis, insufficient water intake, drainage or suction, use of concentrated infant formula
6. (Table 2.3) Signs and symptoms include sunken, soft eyes; decreased skin turgor; thirst, weight loss; rapid, weak pulse and low blood pressure; fatigue, weakness, dizziness, and possible stupor; increased body temperature. The most serious problems are decreased BP and potential shock.
7. increasing thirst, falling blood pressure (BP), increasing heart rate, constricting cutaneous blood vessels, and decreasing urinary output
8. Dehydration is a more serious problem for infants and elderly people, who lack significant fluid reserves as well as the ability to conserve fluid quickly. Infants also experience not only greater insensible water losses through their proportionately larger body surface area but also an increased need for water, owing to their higher metabolic rate.
9. Third-spacing refers to a situation in which fluid shifts out of the blood into a body cavity or tissue where it is no longer available as circulating fluid. Examples include peritonitis, or inflammation and infection of the peritoneal membranes, and burns.

ELECTROLYTE IMBALANCES

10.
    i. hyponatremia, hyperkalemia, hypocalcemia, hypermagnesemia, hyperphosphatemia
    ii. hyponatremia, hypochloremia
    iii. hypernatremia, hyperchloremia
    iv. hypernatremia, hypokalemia, hyperchloremia
    v. hypercalcemia, hypophosphatemia, hypomagnesemia
    vi. hyponatremia, hypochloremia
    vii. hypercalcemia
    viii. hyponatremia, hypokalemia, hypomagnesemia (with potassium-sparing diuretics: hyperkalemia)
    ix. hyponatremia, hyperkalemia, hypochloremia
    x. hypocalcemia
    xi. hypercalcemia
    xii. hyponatremia, hypokalemia, hypophosphatemia
11. skeletal muscle spasm due to hypocalcemia
12. (Table 2.6) hypokalemia and hyperkalemia; (Table 2.7) hypocalcemia and hypercalcemia
13. (Table 2.7) hypercalcemia
14. (Table 2.5) Hyponatremia impairs nerve conduction, causing fatigue, cramps, and seizures, and shifts fluid into cells, leading to hypovolemia. Hypernatremia shifts fluid out of cells, causing cell shrinkage and symptoms like weakness and agitation.
15. PTH raises serum calcium by increasing bone resorption, intestinal absorption (via vitamin D), and renal calcium reabsorption. Calcitonin lowers calcium by inhibiting bone resorption. Vitamin D enhances intestinal calcium absorption.

ACID-BASE IMBALANCES

16. Normal serum pH range is 7.35 to 7.45. pH less than 6.8 and greater than 7.8 usually results in death.
17. Three mechanisms controlling pH are buffer systems, the respiratory system, and the renal system.
18. 20:1
19. sodium bicarbonate—carbonic acid system; phosphate system; hemoglobin system; protein system
20. The respiratory system compensates by increasing the respiratory rate to expel more CO_2 (acid) when hydrogen ions or CO_2 rise, or decreasing the rate to retain CO_2 during alkalosis.
21. The kidneys compensate by excreting hydrogen ions and reabsorbing bicarbonate to reduce acidity in acidosis, or retaining hydrogen ions and excreting bicarbonate to increase acidity in alkalosis, adjusting urine pH from 4.5 to 8.
22. (Table 2.9 and Fig. 2.12)
    i. respiratory acidosis—more acidic urine
    ii. metabolic alkalosis—slow, shallow respirations and increased pH of urine
    iii. respiratory acidosis—more acidic urine
    iv. metabolic acidosis—increased renal excretion of acids and conservation of bicarbonate
    v. respiratory alkalosis—less acidic urine
    vi. respiratory acidosis—more acidic urine and increased rate and depth of respiration (if possible)
    vii. metabolic acidosis—increased rate and depth of respirations, more acidic urine
    viii. metabolic acidosis—increased rate and depth of respiration

TREATMENT OF IMBALANCES

23. Treat the underlying cause, replace deficits (e.g., fluids, electrolytes like sodium/potassium, or bicarbonate for acidosis), or remove excesses (e.g., via diuretics for fluid overload). Monitor electrolyte levels to maintain balance during treatment.

CHAPTER 3: Introduction to Basic Pharmacology and Other Common Therapies

1. circulation and cardiovascular function; age; gender; body weight and proportion of fatty tissue; activity level; liver and kidney function; food and fluid intake; genetic factors; presence of chronic or acute disease

Copyright © 2027 by Elsevier, Inc. All rights are reserved, including those for text and data mining, AI training, and similar technologies.

2. Dose is the amount of drug administered at a single time; dosage is the total amount of the drug given over a period of time.
3. Therapeutic effect is the desired action; adverse (severe) or side (mild) effects are the unwanted or undesirable effects.
4. hypersensitivity (allergic reactions; see Chapter 7 Type I allergic reactions); idiosyncratic reactions: unexpected or unusual responses to drugs; iatrogenic reactions: negative effect due to medication error, drug overdose, unusual response; teratogenic/harmful effects on the fetus; drug interactions: effect of drug is modified when combined with another drug, food, herbal compounds, or other materials
5.
   i. applied to the skin or mucous membranes (e.g., steroid cream, local anesthetics, antimicrobials, eye drops)
   ii. patch applied to the skin for absorption into the blood (e.g., long-term continuous administration of nitroglycerin, nicotine patch, scopolamine patch, estradiol)
   iii. by mouth (e.g., aspirin, vitamins, cough syrup, antibiotics)
   iv. under the tongue (e.g., nitroglycerin, loperamide, testosterone)
   v. injection beneath the epidermis and dermis, into the subcutaneous layer of the skin (e.g., insulin, heparin, interferon)
   vi. injection into the muscle (e.g., penicillin, meperidine, tetanus and diphtheria toxoid, vitamin B_{12})
   vii. injection into a vein, into the bloodstream (e.g., general anesthetic like sodium pentothal, morphine, diazepam, vincristine)
   viii. into the respiratory tract (e.g., bronchodilator medication, glucocorticoid inhaler, anesthetics such as nitrous oxide)
6. topical
7.

	Onset of Action	Advantages	Disadvantages
Topical	Rapid	Easy to apply	Can be messy, smelly, or unpleasant
Transdermal	Rapid; long-term, continuous	Easy to apply for long-term, continuous administration	Action may continue after desired effect achieved
Oral	Long time to onset (30–60 min)	Tablets, capsules, stable, variable cost but relatively inexpensive; self-administered	Taste and swallowing problems; gastric irritation; uncertain absorption due to food interactions
Sublingual	Immediate	Rapid and prolonged effect; can be administered to unconscious patient	Tablets are soft and unstable over time
Subcutaneous	Slow absorption; some drug loss	Simplest injection; only small doses may be given	Requires training, asepsis, and equipment; may be irritating
Intramuscular	Good absorption into blood, sometimes lag and drug loss	Rapid, prolonged effect; can be used when patient unconscious or nauseated	Requires training, asepsis, and equipment; short shelf-life; some injection discomfort
Intravenous	Immediate and no drug loss	Immediate effect; predictable drug levels; can be used when patient unconscious	Costly; injection skill required; drug irritation at the IV site
Inhalation	Rapid; little loss of drug	Local effect or absorbed into alveolar capillaries; rapid; good for anesthesia	Requires training in effective technique

8. intravenous, sublingual, inhalation and topical, subcutaneous, intramuscular, oral
9. Once in the bloodstream, drugs are transported by the circulating blood through various pathways, branching off into different organs or tissues. Depending on the specific characteristics of a drug, some may be lost temporarily in storage areas such as fatty tissue (e.g., anesthetics) or may be quickly metabolized. Eventually, the drug reaches the target organ or tissue, moves into the interstitial fluid, and exerts its effect. Most drugs are gradually metabolized and inactivated in the liver and then excreted in the kidneys—a few in the bile or feces.
10. Drugs interact with natural specific tissue receptors and act by either (a) stimulating the receptors, increasing biological activity; or (b) blocking the receptor sites, decreasing activity.

Copyright © 2027 by Elsevier, Inc. All rights are reserved, including those for text and data mining, AI training, and similar technologies.

11. Drugs are removed from the circulation in the liver, where they are absorbed by the cells whose various metabolic pathways catabolize them.
12. by the kidneys
13. Disease of the liver could impair or slow drug metabolism; therefore, the drug is active longer. This prolongs the drug's effects. If the individual is taking the drug regularly, blood levels will gradually increase, possibly resulting in toxic effects. Liver disease may result in decreased production of plasma proteins. This results in decreased protein binding, resulting in increased free drug in circulation and therefore increased drug effects. Kidney disease may interfere with drug excretion—the drug and its metabolites could accumulate, resulting in increased and prolonged drug effects.
14. Inhalation anesthetics are generally excreted via the lungs; it would be difficult to predict the individual's response. There would be problems assessing both the dosage and the rate of drug removal. Intravenous anesthetics depress the respiratory center. This could cause additional hypoxia and increase the risk of developing acidosis.
15.
    i. newborns and babies: immature liver and drug effects more difficult to predict; also have much smaller body mass elderly: may have diseases that interfere with drug metabolism and excretion; also more likely to be taking more than one medication, increasing the possibility of drug interactions
    ii. Smaller individuals require less medication—for children, generally the dosage is calculated according to body weight.
    iii. Pregnant women should avoid drug usage whenever possible because many drugs cross the placenta and may cause teratogenic effects.
    Breastfeeding women should also avoid drug use because many drugs are excreted, to some degree, in milk and can affect the child.
    Gender differences—metabolism, percentage body fat, percentage body fluids
    iv. If an individual believes a drug is going to be effective, this will likely have a positive effect; the converse is true. Positive suggestion or reinforcement therefore are often useful "placebo" effects.
    v. Heart disease may impair circulation, resulting in decreased distribution, metabolism, and excretion of drugs.
    Liver disease could impair or slow drug metabolism. Therefore the drug is active longer—this prolongs the drug's effects. If the individual is taking the drug regularly, blood levels will gradually increase, possibly resulting in toxic effects. Liver disease may result in decreased production of plasma proteins. This results in decreased protein binding, resulting in increased free drug in circulation and therefore increased drug effects. Kidney disease may interfere with drug excretion. Therefore the drug and its metabolites could accumulate, resulting in increased and prolonged drug effects.
    vi. Some medications should be taken with food, whereas others must be taken on an empty stomach to prevent food interactions. Therefore it is important to always confirm with a pharmacist, nurse, or physician.
    Certain drugs should not be taken at bedtime, e.g., diuretics (water pills, stimulants).
    Antibiotics should be evenly spaced throughout the day.
    vii. determines onset of action; also determines whether there may be drug destruction (e.g., oral route—drug may be destroyed by gastric pH or by food)
    viii. Generally, the higher the dosage is, the greater the therapeutic effect will be. Unfortunately, as dosage increases, so do the incidence and severity of adverse and even toxic effects.
    ix. This will determine onset and duration of action (e.g., liquids are absorbed faster than pills; enteric coating delays onset and may prolong duration of action).
    x. Is the client taking the drug at the prescribed times, with or without food?
    xi. A quiet, stress-free environment enhances the effectiveness of analgesics by helping the individual relax.
    If someone has just vomited, removing the emesis and opening the window to improve ventilation will enhance the effectiveness of the antiemetic.
    xii. These may enhance or decrease drug action (e.g., ingestion of alcohol potentiates narcotics, hypnotics, and sedatives, and caffeine will antagonize hypnotics and sedatives).
16.
    i. allergic, immunological reaction; e.g., penicillin allergy
    ii. unexpected or unusual responses to drugs; e.g., excessive excitement after administration of a sedative
    iii. in which one drug enhances the action of another; e.g., epinephrine enhances the effects of local anesthetic without increasing the dose
    iv. the effect of a combination of drugs is much greater than expected; e.g., combination of drugs to treat pain
    v. the effects of a combination of drugs are greatly decreased; e.g., antidotes for poisoning
    vi. when the body adapts to a drug, over time, resulting in a higher dosage to achieve the desired effect, e.g., use of narcotic analgesia
    vii. therapeutic effects after administration of a substance that does not have the pharmacological effects of the drug being studied; e.g., use in research study
17. Generic names are unique, official, simple names for specific drugs; chemical names reflect the often-complex chemical structure of the drug.

Copyright © 2027 by Elsevier, Inc. All rights are reserved,
including those for text and data mining, AI training, and similar technologies.

18. mind-body therapies, biologically based therapies, manipulative and body-based methods, energy therapies, whole medical systems
19.
   i. individualized treatment and rehabilitation to restore function as well as reduce pain, involving various modalities including exercises, ultrasound, and transcutaneous electrical nerve stimulation (TENS)
   ii. assessment and treatment of communication or swallowing disorders
   iii. functional assessment and treatments to restore activities of daily living (ADLs)
   iv. use of plant, animal, and mineral products to stimulate the immune system and natural healing power of the body
   v. medical practice using surgery and drugs in addition to manipulations of the musculoskeletal system to promote healing
   vi. use of essential oils from plants that have therapeutic effects when applied topically or inhaled
   vii. therapy that frequently involves manipulation of the vertebral column—no drugs or surgery
   viii. use of techniques to increase circulation, reduce pain, increase flexibility, and reduce muscle spasm
   ix. Uses EEG to measure/monitor brain waves, ECG to measure/monitor heart rate and EMG to measure/monitor muscle contractions
20. Acupuncture involves the use of needles inserted into acupoints on the body; it is designed to balance the life energy in the body. Imbalances of these life energies are thought to be responsible for disease. Shiatsu is a massage therapy designed to apply pressure to acupoints, rather than inserting needles into acupoints, in an effort to bring balance to the life energies. Yoga involves the combining of physical activity in the form of stretching postures with meditation to improve the flow of life energy throughout the body.
21. U.S. Food and Drug Administration

CHAPTER 4: Pain

1. inflammation, infection, ischemia, tissue necrosis, stretching of tissue, chemicals, burns
2. Somatic pain arises from skin or deeper structures (*i.e.,* bone or muscle); visceral pain originates in the organs.
3. bradykinin, histamine, prostaglandin
4. (Fig. 4.1)
   - Stimulation of pain receptors (nociceptors) by thermal, chemical, or physical stimuli
     If the stimulus exceeds the *threshold* of the receptors, the associated nerve fibers transmit a "pain" signal to the spinal cord and brain.
   - Myelinated A delta fibers (acute pain) or unmyelinated C fibers (chronic pain) transmit the afferent pain impulse to the dorsal root ganglia and then to the spinal cord.
   - Sensory impulse reaches the spinal cord synapse and from there crosses over to the opposite spinothalamic tract (neospinothalamic tract for acute sharp pain; paleospinothalamic tract for chronic or dull pain). [Reflex response to sudden pain at the spinal cord level results in involuntary muscle contraction to move the body part away from the source of pain.]
   - The impulse moves up the lateral spinothalamic tract to the reticular formation (influencing brain awareness) in the brainstem, the hypothalamus (stress response), the thalamus, and other structures (limbic system; emotional response) as they ascend to the somatic sensory area of the cerebral cortex and the parietal lobe of the brain, where the location and character of the pain are perceived.
5. (Fig. 4.2) Endorphins (enkephalins, dynorphin, beta-lipotropins) are released by interneurons of the spinal cord; they then attach to opiate receptors and block the release of substance P.
6. (Fig. 4.3) Referred pain occurs when pain is perceived at a site distant from the source. It is due to multiple sensory fibers from different sources connecting at a single level of the spinal cord, making it difficult for the brain to discern the actual origin of the pain. An example is the pain of a heart attack, which is experienced in the left neck and/or arm. Pain in the shoulder may also occur.
7. Acute pain is generally sudden, severe, and short term. Chronic (long-term) pain is more difficult to treat, and prognosis may be less certain.
8. (Tables 4.2 and 4.3) Pain can be managed in a number of ways. The most common method of management is use of analgesic medications to relieve pain. Sedatives and antianxiety drugs are often used to promote rest and relaxation. Using them in conjunction with analgesics may reduce the dosage of pain medication required. Severe pain may be self-managed by the patient through use of patient-controlled analgesia (PCA). A small pump attached to a vascular access site allows the patient to medicate as needed and reduces the overall amount of narcotic needed. Other methods for managing pain include stress reduction and relaxation, distractors, heat and cold applications, massage, physiotherapy, exercise, therapeutic touch, hypnosis imaging, and acupuncture, which may modify the brain's pain perception and response. Finally, surgical intervention may be necessary to sever the sensory nerve pathway. Injections may be used to achieve similar effects.
9. Pain relief for conditions such as myofascial pain syndrome, fibromyalgia, headaches.
   Substances that may be used are:
   Local anesthetics, blocking pain receptors in muscles
   Corticosteroids, reducing inflammation
   Botulinum toxin A, interferes with nerve signaling pathways and prevents muscle contraction
10. age, culture, family traditions, and prior experience

Copyright © 2027 by Elsevier, Inc. All rights reserved, including those for text and data mining, AI training, and similar technologies.

11. (Table 4.2)

	Nonnarcotic Analgesics	Narcotic Analgesics
Action	Decrease pain at peripheral site; all are antipyretic; ASA and NSAIDs are also antiinflammatory	1. Codeine and oxycodone: act on opiate receptors in the CNS and affect pain perception 2. Morphine and meperidine: act on CNS, producing euphoria and sedation; block pain pathways in the spinal cord and brain
Adverse effects	Nausea, gastric ulcers, bleeding, allergies	1. Nausea, constipation, and, at higher doses, respiratory depression 2. Addiction
Uses	For mild pain, especially when inflammation is present	1. Moderate pain 2. Severe pain
Examples	Tylenol, ibuprofen, naproxen, aspirin	1. Codeine, alone or in combination with acetaminophen; oxycodone 2. Morphine; meperidine

ASA, acetylsalicylic acid (aspirin); *CNS,* central nervous system; *NSAIDs,* nonsteroidal antiinflammatory drugs.

12. (Table 4.3)
Local anesthesia: injected or topical; lidocaine, blocks nerve conduction; removal of skin lesion, tooth extraction
Spinal or regional anesthesia: local anesthetic into subarachnoid or epidural space; blocks nerve conduction (sensation) below the level of injection; labor and delivery
General anesthesia: intravenous (thiopental) or inhalation (nitrous oxide); loss of consciousness; general surgery
13. myelinated A delta fibers: fibers are wrapped in myelin sheath and transmit impulses very rapidly. Associated with the acute pain.
Unmyelinated C fibers: no myelin sheath, transmit impulses slowly. Associated with chronic pain.
14. The gate-control theory posits that "gates" at spinal cord synapses can modulate pain signals, either allowing or blocking their transmission to the brain. Pain impulses are inhibited when gates close due to competing sensory stimuli (e.g., touch) or brain signals releasing endorphins, which block substance P release. Practical applications include transcutaneous electrical nerve stimulation (TENS), massage, acupuncture, and distraction techniques, which stimulate nonpain pathways or increase endorphin release to reduce pain perception.

CHAPTER 5: Inflammation and Healing

1. mechanical barrier such as intact skin and mucous membrane
2. second: processes of phagocytosis and inflammation; third: the immune system response
3. The immune system is the specific defense mechanism of the body. It provides protection by stimulating a unique response following exposure to foreign substances. (See also review of the immune system in Chapter 7.)
4. (Fig. 5.2) process by which neutrophils, monocytes, and macrophages engulf and destroy bacteria, cellular debris, or foreign material
5. Inflammation is the body's nonspecific response to injury that involves increased blood flow to the area to localize and remove an injurious agent. Inflammation can cause redness, swelling, warmth, and pain; loss of function is also possible. It may be caused by direct physical damage such as cuts or sprains, caustic chemicals such as acids or drain cleaners, ischemia or infarction, allergic reactions, extremes of heat or cold, foreign bodies such as splinters or glass, and infection.
6. The two main events are vasodilation, and increased capillary permeability in response to a chemical mediator (e.g., histamine, serotonin, etc.) released at the site of injury. This allows for the accumulation in the area of fluid (to dilute any toxic substances) and specific plasma proteins such as globulins or antibodies (to react with specific antigens) and fibrinogen (to form a fibrin mesh to localize the problem).
7. Redness, heat, swelling and pain" Redness and heat due to increased blood flow, swelling due to shift of protein and fluid into interstitial space, pain due to increased pressure of fluid on the nerves.
8. Events of the cellular response:
chemotaxis
margination
emigration (diapedesis)
phagocytosis and subsequent release of lysosomal enzymes
9. (Table 5.2)
a. vii
b. iii
c. ii, v
d. i
e. vii and viii
f. vi
g. vi
h. i, iv, vi

Copyright © 2027 by Elsevier, Inc. All rights are reserved, including those for text and data mining, AI training, and similar technologies.

10. fever due to the release of pyrogens by leukocytes and macrophages; malaise, fatigue, headache, and anorexia
11. infection in inflamed tissue, deep ulcers (from severe or prolonged inflammation), skeletal muscle spasms or strong muscle contractions, local complications such as tissue destruction and scarring, immobility due to pain or edema (edema compresses organs such as blood vessels and airways)
12. (Fig. 5.5)

Characteristic	Acute Inflammation	Chronic Inflammation
Causative agents	Direct damage (trauma) Chemicals Ischemia Cell necrosis or infarction Allergic reactions Physical agents (burns) Foreign bodies (splinters or dirt) Infection	When the cause persists and is not removed or eradicated
Signs and symptoms	Immediate or occurring within a few hours (e.g., sunburn) Severity varies with the situation or cause	Delayed and prolonged over a significant period of time (may be intermittent) Severity varies depending on the cause and pathophysiology and duration
Cells involved	Neutrophils and macrophages; lymphocytes if an immune response is involved	Lymphocytes, macrophages, fibroblasts
Treatment	Acetaminophen, glucocorticoids and NSAIDs, RICE (rest, ice, compression, elevation)	Acetaminophen, NSAIDs and ACTH, exercise, physiotherapy and pain modification
Results	Healing unless it becomes chronic due to persistence of causative agent; regeneration or resolution	Scarring and/or granuloma Tissue breakdown may occur with bleeding and loss of function

13.
R = Rest allows time for healing, minimizing further pain and irritation to the injured area.
I = Early application of cold causes vasoconstriction, decreasing pain and edema.
C = Compression reduces edema and pain by activating alternate sensory pathways.
E = Elevation improves fluid flow away from the damaged area.
14. NSAIDs are analgesic and antipyretic. They may cause allergic reactions, slow blood clotting, and cause nausea and/or stomach ulceration. Steroids decrease immune responses and increase the risk of infection, hypertension, and edema. They may also cause osteoporosis and skeletal muscle wasting.
15. NSAIDs are antiinflammatory. They may cause allergic reactions and slow blood clotting. Acetaminophen has no antiinflammatory action. Overuse at higher dosages than recommended may cause kidney and liver damage.
16. heat, physiotherapy, adequate nutrition and hydration, mild to moderate exercise, elastic stockings to reduce fluid accumulation.
17. Resolution occurs when there is minimal tissue damage, the damage is repaired, and cells recover and resume normal function in a short time. Regeneration is the healing process that occurs in tissues whose cells are capable of mitosis (e.g., epithelial cells of the skin, gastrointestinal tract). The damaged cells are replaced by the proliferation of nearby undamaged cells.
18. (Boxes 5.1 and 5.2)
    i. Inoperable bullet wound to the brain may be inaccessible without further tissue damage and loss of function.
    ii. Malnutrition, especially deficiencies in vitamins such as C, E, and K, would impair the blood-clotting capability of the individual, impairing wound closure and delaying repair of damaged tissues.
    iii. Large, deep cuts, for example, especially if untreated, or presenting difficult suture closure would facilitate extensive scar formation (e.g., cuts due to broken glass or power tools).
    iv. Anticlotting medications would limit or impair clotting and hence wound closure (e.g., aspirin and other blood-thinning drugs before surgery).
    v. Nutritional status is often inadequate in the very old, and the aging process itself slows down normal healing responses at many levels.
    vi. Foreign bodies, if not removed, impair wound closure and promote scarring as well as predispose to infection (e.g., a large splinter).
    vii. If the blood supply is limited or is absent from the damaged tissue, then most of the cellular and blood factors necessary for healing will not reach the affected area.

Copyright © 2027 by Elsevier, Inc. All rights are reserved, including those for text and data mining, AI training, and similar technologies.

viii. Infection requires its own cure, before healing can occur; removal of the infectious agent, if impaired or delayed, would prolong the healing process, leading to more extensive scarring and, if untreated, perhaps systemic infection. A puncture wound, like a rusty nail, could bring infection to the damaged tissue. Another example is a bite from a rabid animal.
ix. Broken bones, if not immobilized, do not heal properly. (See Chapter 9 for further discussion on fracture healing.)
x. Disease, if chronic and with systemic effects, could impair immune and other normal healing tissue responses. Diabetes, for example, may result in impaired circulation to the damaged area.

19. loss of function; contractures and obstructions; adhesions; hypertrophic scar tissue; ulceration
20. (Figs. 5.10, 5.11, and 5.12)
    i. Partial-thickness burns involve the epidermis and part of the dermis; deep partial-thickness burns involve destruction of the epidermis and part of the dermis; full-thickness burns result in destruction of all skin layers and often underlying subcutaneous tissues as well, fourth degree burns in which both layers of skin are destroyed as well as damage/destruction of deeper lying tissues
    ii. The percentage of body surface area (BSA) burned uses the "rule of nines" for calculation to determine extent of injury and fluid replacement needs.
21. Nerves in the burned area have been destroyed.
22. shock, respiratory problems, pain, infection
23. excision/removal of damaged tissue, antibiotics, covering of wound
24. See Fig. 5.12, Assessment of burn area using the rule of nines
    Total head—9%
    Two arms—18%
    Trunk—36%
    Perineum—1%
    Two legs—36%
25. There is an ongoing need to produce more body heat and replace damaged/destroyed tissue (especially the skin and erythrocytes), which means higher nutrient demands.
26.
    - Turmeric: used for thousands of years in Chinese medicine to treat many inflammatory conditions such as joint pain, arthritis, and stomach issues. The main mechanism seems to be its antioxidant capacity linked to the compound curcumin.
    - Black pepper: its antiinflammatory properties are due to piperine, the active phenolic compound in black pepper.
    - Ginger root: could be a potential substitute for nonsteroidal antiinflammatory drugs.
    - Rosemary: several complex actions in the inflammatory cascade to include the inhibition of cytokine release from activated T-cells.
    - Others: cloves, cayenne pepper, basil, peppermint, cinnamon, sage, coriander, and many more.

CHAPTER 6: Infection

1. Growth factors such as pH, temperature, carbohydrates, and oxygen requirements can determine the site of infection. Example: *Clostridium tetani* is anaerobic and therefore favors deep tissue infections.
2. Inflammation is a normal body response to anything that results in tissue damage. Infection is when microorganisms reproduce in or on body tissues.

BACTERIA

3. (Fig. 6.1): A: coccus, B: bacillus, C: vibrio, D: spirilla, E: pleiomorphic, F: spirochete, G: diplo-, H: staph(ylo)-, I: strep(to)-, J: palisades, K: tetrad
4. (Fig. 6.3) The basic structure of a bacterium consists of an outer rigid cell wall, a cell membrane, a DNA strand, and cytoplasm. In addition, some species contain an external capsule or slime layer, specialized structures such as flagella, and pili or fimbriae.
5. Gram-positive bacteria have a thick peptidoglycan layer in the cell wall—they stain purple with the standard Gram stain process. Gram-negative have a very thin peptidoglycan layer, and they stain red/pink in the Gram stain process.
6. Exotoxins are produced/secreted by Gram-positive bacteria. Endotoxins are components of the cell wall of Gram-negative organisms.
7. (Figs. 6.5 and 6.6) Endospores are latent forms of some bacterial species with an outer coat that is resistant to heat and other environmental conditions. The process of spore formation is illustrated in Fig. 6.6. Examples of spore-producing bacteria include tetanus *(C. tetani)* and botulism *(C. botulinum)*.
8. (Fig. 6.6) Binary fission is simply dividing in half, forming two daughter cells identical to the parent bacterium.
9. (Table 6.2)

	Bacterial Cells	**Human (Eukaryotic) Cells**
Cell wall	Present	Not present
Cell membrane	Present—selectively permeable; site of metabolic processes	Present—selectively permeable
Capsule or slime coat	Present in some	Not present

Copyright © 2027 by Elsevier, Inc. All rights are reserved, including those for text and data mining, AI training, and similar technologies.

	Bacterial Cells	Human (Eukaryotic) Cells
Flagella	Present	Sperm only
Pili or fimbriae	Present in some	Not present
Cilia	Not present	Present in some
Membrane-bound organelles (mitochondria, lysosomes, endoplasmic reticulum)	Not present	Present
Ribosomes	Present	Present—larger
Nucleus	Not present	Present
Number of chromosomes	Single; circular	46; paired (except sex cells)
Method of reproduction	Binary fission	Mitosis

VIRUSES

10. They require a living host cell for replication.
11. (Fig. 6.1*B*) The virion consists of a protein coat or capsid and a DNA or RNA nucleic acid core.
12. (Fig. 6.7) Virus attaches to the host cell and penetrates. It uncoats and takes over the host cell DNA. The host cell synthesizes viral components. The components assemble and are released by host cell lysis. Sometimes the virus may remain inactive in the host cell or activate at a later time.

FUNGI

13. (Figs. 6.1*C* and 7.16*C*) Fungi are classified as eukaryotic. They consist of cells or chains of cells and may have long filaments called hyphae that intertwine to form a mass called the mycelium, which is large enough to be visible.
14. (Table 6.2)

	Bacteria	Fungi	Virus
Basic structure	Cell wall, cell membrane, cytoplasm, DNA	Cell wall, hyphae Eukaryotic	Capsid, nucleic acid core of either RNA or DNA
Method of reproduction	Binary fission	Budding, spores, extending hyphae	Uses host cell to replicate and assemble components
Method of culturing	Various culture media	Culture media (simple glucose/agar)	Living host cells
Drugs used to treat	Antimicrobials	Antifungal agents	Antiviral drugs

OTHER MICROORGANISMS

15.
    i. chlamydiae: pelvic inflammatory disease; eye infections in newborn of infected mothers
    ii. rickettsiae: typhus; Rocky Mountain spotted fever
    iii. mycoplasmas: pneumonia
    iv. protozoa: *Trichomonas vaginalis;* malaria; amoebic dysentery
16. Helminths are round or flat worms. Examples include tape worm and hook worm.
17. Prions are proteinaceous agents that are transmitted by the consumption of contaminated tissue. They cause Creutzfeldt-Jakob disease in humans.
18. microorganisms that normally inhabit various areas of the body, such as the skin and gastrointestinal tract
19. (Table 6.3) Brain, blood, kidneys, bladder
20. Endemic infections are those that consistently occur in a population.
21. A pandemic is an infectious disease that has spread worldwide (a worldwide epidemic). Pandemics in the last 100 years are: Spanish flu (1918); Asian flu (1957); Hong Kong flu (1968); Human Immunodeficiency Virus (HIV—1981 and ongoing); Swine flu (2009); COVID-19 (2019 and ongoing). The most current is the COVID-19 pandemic, and measures have been taken unlike with any other pandemic. These include shutdown of businesses, schools, universities and other educational institutions, banning gatherings of people not living in the same household, restricted travel, and more. Wearing of protective face masks and keeping distance from other people is mandatory in many countries. Furthermore, testing is required in many situations. Vaccination is ongoing.
22. Pathogenicity is the capacity of a microbe to cause disease. Virulence is the degree of pathogenicity of a

Copyright © 2027 by Elsevier, Inc. All rights reserved, including those for text and data mining, AI training, and similar technologies.

microbe or pathogen. It can be enhanced by production of exotoxins or endotoxins, destructive enzymes, spore formation, and presence of bacterial capsules. Immunodeficiency or immunodepression can result in opportunistic infections; relocation of normal flora to another body site can also result in the production of disease.

CONSOLIDATION OF MICROBIOLOGY

23.
   i. fungi
   ii. fungi
   iii. bacteria
   iv. protozoa
   v. bacteria
   vi. bacteria; viruses; fungi
   vii. bacteria
   viii. rickettsiae
   ix. fungi
   x. viruses
   xi. viruses
   xii. bacteria

CONTROL OF TRANSMISSION AND INFECTION

24. Disinfectants are designed for use on nonliving surfaces; antiseptics are designed to be used on living tissue.
25. (Fig. 6.14) The components and means to break the cycle include locating and removing the reservoir or sources of infection; blocking the exit from the source; providing or cleaning/sterilizing barriers; maintaining immunizations; and treating or quarantining infection or carrier.
26. (Fig. 6.17) The disk diffusion method involves plating a small amount of the specimen to produce a bacterial colony and placing paper disks impregnated with an antibiotic on the inoculated plate. After a 24-hour incubation, if there is a clear zone of inhibition surrounding the disk, the zone will be measured to determine the effectiveness of the agent. If there is no zone, the bacteria are resistant to the antibiotic. The Minimum Inhibitory Concentration method uses a series of dilutions of an antimicrobial agent applied against a known pathogen to determine the minimum concentration of a specific agent that is effective against the organism.
27.
   i. the range of bacteria for which the drug is effective: narrow, either Gram-positive or Gram-negative; broad, both Gram-positive and Gram-negative bacteria
   ii. bacteria that develop or adapt so as to lose their sensitivity to a drug, such as altering their metabolism to block the drug's effects, producing enzymes that inactivate the drug, altering their cell membranes
   iii. drugs that kill microorganisms
   iv. drugs that inhibit bacterial reproduction
28. a secondary or new infection by pathogens that results from disruption or reduction of the normal resident flora by antimicrobial drugs
29. allergic reactions, anaphylaxis, disruption of resident flora, secondary infections
30. A superinfection occurs only during treatment with antimicrobial agents. An opportunistic infection occurs in an individual with decreased immunity. Both are usually caused by fungi or bacteria that are part of the normal resident flora or when resident flora from one area of the body is introduced to another area causing an infection there.
31. when the identity of the bacterium is known; after culture and sensitivity have been completed
32. The drug prevents replication of the bacteria, thereby keeping the number of bacteria constant—the body's own defensive cells will destroy the organism.
33. if the individual was immunosuppressed (e.g., organ transplant recipient) or immunodeficient (e.g., someone with AIDS)
34. Bacteria adapt and/or mutate to develop various means of losing drug sensitivity; excessive or unnecessary use of drugs provides a stimulus for such adaptation.
35. because they may reduce the risk of secondary bacterial infection
36. The drug should be taken regularly according to the prescription. The drug should be taken until the prescription is completely used. Follow instructions regarding food or fluid intake. Provide a good medical history, including known drug allergies.
37. Because viruses are obligate intracellular parasites, a drug that destroys viruses would also destroy the host cell.
38. Interferons enhance nearby cells' resistance to viral infection and inhibit viral replication. They also stimulate the immune system, reducing viral spread. In treatment, interferons are used for conditions like cancer, though their efficacy for widespread disease management is limited.
39. Septicemia triggers a toxic inflammatory response, leading to systemic symptoms like fever, fatigue, confusion, and seizures. It increases capillary permeability, causing fluid loss, shock, and potential organ failure.

CHAPTER 7: Immunity

1. The three main components of the immune system are: lymphoid tissue, immune cells, and tissues concerned with immune cell development. Lymphoid tissue: lymph nodes, spleen, tonsils, intestinal lymphoid tissue, lymphatic circulation. Immune cells: lymphocytes, macrophages. Cell development: bone marrow, thymus gland.
2. See Fig. 7.1 Structures in the immune system
   A. Pharyngeal tonsil (Adenoid)
   B. Palatine tonsil
   C. Lymph nodes—cervical
   D. Lymphatic vessels
   E. Lymph nodes—axillary
   F. Spleen
   G. Lymph nodes—intestinal
   H. Lymph nodes—inguinal

Copyright © 2027 by Elsevier, Inc. All rights are reserved,
including those for text and data mining, AI training, and similar technologies.

I. Bone marrow
J. Thymus

3. A cell surface antigen is a unique protein or glycoprotein configuration that is a distinctive marker for the recognition of a cell by the immune system. It provides the means by which the immune system distinguishes self from "nonself". It is important because it provides for the detection and identification of nonself by the immune system. This differentiation underlies the host defense against infection and other foreign antigens, and it forms the basis for selection of compatible organs and tissues for transplantation.
4. The major histocompatibility complex (MHC) cell membrane antigens are molecules that are specific for each individual. The HLA is the human MHC on human leukocytes that determine "self" and serve as the basis for identifying histocompatible cells and tissues for transplantation, including blood transfusion. These antigens representing "self" are present on an individual's cell membranes.
5. (Table 7.1 and Chapter 5, Table 5.1)

Chemical Mediator	Source	Effects
Histamine	Mast cells and basophils	Vasodilation and increased vascular permeability, contraction of bronchiolar smooth muscle; pruritus
Prostaglandins	Group of lipids synthesized in mast cells	Various effects from causing inflammation, vasodilation, increased capillary permeability, muscle spasm, and pain
Cytokines (lymphokines, monokines, interleukins, interferon)	T lymphocytes and macrophages	Increase in plasma proteins, Erythrocyte Sedimentation Rate ESR; stimulate activation and proliferation of B and T cells and communication between cells (messengers); induce fever, leukocytosis, and chemotaxis
Leukotrienes	Group of lipids derived from mast cells and basophils	Contraction of bronchiolar smooth muscle; vasodilation and increased capillary permeability; chemotaxis
Kinins (bradykinin)	Activation of plasma protein (kinogen [e.g., bradykinin])	Vasodilation, edema, and pain
Complement	Group of proteins circulating in the bloodstream; activated by antigen-antibody reactions on cell surface	Release of chemical mediators, promoting inflammation, chemotaxis, phagocytosis, cell membrane damage (e.g., hemolysis)

6. (Table 7.1; see also Table 5.1)
   i. histamine, prostaglandins, kinins, leukotrienes
   ii. histamine, prostaglandins, leukotrienes
   iii. cytokines, leukotrienes, complement
   iv. prostaglandins, kinins
   v. histamine, leukotrienes
   vi. cytokines
   vii. histamine
   viii. tumor necrosis factor (TNF), cytokines
7. (Table 7.1)
   Macrophages: phagocytosis; foreign antigen recognition
   Natural killer (NK) cells: destroy foreign cells, virus-infected cells, and cancer cells
   T lymphocytes: stimulated by particular antigen to initiate cell mediated immune response
   Cytotoxic or killer T cells: destroy antigens and cancer and virus-infected cells
   Helper T cells (T4 or CD4): activate B and T cells; limit immune response
   Memory T cells: remember antigen and stimulate immune response upon subsequent exposure (secondary response)
   Suppressor T cells (T8): limit immune response
   B lymphocytes: stimulated by particular antigen cloning becoming plasma cells producing antibodies. A population of cells remains as memory cells following simulation by the antigen.
   Plasma cells: produce specific antibody
   B memory cells: secondary antibody response
8. (Fig. 7.2) helper T cells
9. (Table 7.2) A, B, C: IgG, IgD, IgE (in any order), D: IgA, E: IgM
   IgG: primary and secondary antibody responses; activates complement; includes antibacterials, antivirals, and antitoxins; crosses placenta, creates passive immunity in newborns
   IgM: primary antibody responses; activates complement; forms natural antibodies; is involved in blood ABO incompatibility reactions
   IgA: found in secretions such as tears and saliva, in mucous membranes, and in colostrum to provide protection for newborns
   IgE: binds to mast cells in skin and mucous membranes; when linked to allergen, causes release of histamine and other chemicals, resulting in inflammation
   IgD: attached to B cells; activates B cells

Copyright © 2027 by Elsevier, Inc. All rights are reserved, including those for text and data mining, AI training, and similar technologies.

10. Antibodies exert their effect by binding to the specific antigen that elicited their production, usually on a cell or bacterial surface, resulting in antigen destruction, cell membrane damage (especially in the presence of complement), and, in the case of red blood cells, cell lysis. Some antigen-antibody-complement complexes are also chemotactic, attracting phagocytes and other cells to the site.
11. Primary response on initial antigen exposure may range from days to weeks. Secondary response is almost immediate.
12. (Fig. 7.3) Primary response is approximately 3 to 4 weeks. Secondary response is quicker, with much higher titer within a week or two.
13. mRNA coded to produce a specific protein antigen is taken in by a cell that produces the antigen and presents it on the cell surface, which triggers the immune response providing an immune memory to attack this antigen in potential subsequent infections.
14. A cytokine storm is a physiological reaction by the immune system, causing an uncontrolled and excessive release of cytokines. Cytokine storms can be triggered by both various infectious and noninfectious agents, but especially by viral infections.
15. to promote a stronger, faster secondary immune response by "reminding" the immune system of the previously encountered antigen
16. There are many strains of a virus or bacteria that cause a disease, and they may mutate readily, causing new strains; then, because the immune response is specific, infection with one strain does not create immunity to subsequent exposures to new, different strains.
17. (see Table 7.3)

Characteristic	Active Immunity	Passive Immunity
Method of acquisition	Exposure to antigen and production of specific antibodies	Receiving specific antibody passively (*i.e.,* produced by others who have been exposed to the antigens) via either milk (newborn infants) or injection of pooled IgG fractions
Onset of immunity after exposure to antigen	Several weeks for a primary response	Immediate upon receipt of the antibodies
Duration of effectiveness	Depending on the nature of the antigen, usually lasts for years (memory T cells)	Months
Examples	Polio, measles, diphtheria, vaccines, chickenpox	Breast milk, rabies immune globulin, and snake antivenom serum

18. A close match of HLAs between donor and host tissues reduces risk of rejection. The common treatment involves immunosuppressive drugs, such as cyclosporine, azathioprine (Imuran), and prednisone. The use of tissues that lack a blood supply decreases the potential for rejection.
19. The term *opportunistic* describes microorganisms that are usually harmless in healthy individuals unless conditions occur that favor the growth of the organism over the normal flora. Patients taking immunosuppressant drugs have limited body defenses that are not prepared for an infection by normally harmless organisms.
20. Preventive (prophylactic) antibiotics are usually administered because opportunistic infections are common, can be difficult to treat, and are best prevented.

HYPERSENSITIVITY

21. (Table 7.5)

Type	Mechanism	Effects	Example
I	IgE bound to mast cells; release of histamine and chemical mediators	Immediate inflammation and pruritus	Hay fever, seasonal allergies; anaphylaxis
II	IgG or IgM reacts with antigen on cell—complement activated	Cell lysis and phagocytosis	ABO blood incompatibility
III	Antigen-antibody complex deposits in tissue—complement activated	Inflammation; vasculitis	Autoimmune disorders: systemic lupus erythematosus (SLE); glomerulonephritis
IV	Antigen binds to T lymphocyte; sensitizing lymphocytes that releases lymphokines	Delayed inflammation	Contact dermatitis; transplant rejection

Copyright © 2027 by Elsevier, Inc. All rights are reserved,
including those for text and data mining, AI training, and similar technologies.

22. (Fig. 7.5; see also Chapter 12)

	Hypovolemic Shock	Anaphylactic Shock
Etiology	Hemorrhage, severe burns, dehydration, peritonitis, pancreatitis	Severe, life-threatening, systemic hypersensitivity (allergic) reaction caused by insect stings, ingestion of nuts or shellfish, penicillin, or local anesthetics
Distinguishing features	Anxiety, restlessness, thirst early; tachycardia; cool, pale, moist skin; oliguria; hyperventilation during compensation Progressive: lethargy, weakness, faintness; metabolic acidosis; CNS depression; organ damage	Very rapid onset of decreased blood pressure, weakness, fainting; itching; airway obstruction, cough, dyspnea; edema around the face, hands, and feet; hives, urticaria, fear, and panic. If untreated, collapse and loss of consciousness ensue.
Specific treatment	Put patient in supine position; cover to keep warm; call for help or transport to hospital. Administer oxygen, whole blood, plasma, or fluids with electrolytes, if available and ordered.	Epinephrine injection immediately; oxygen administration; antihistamine injection; treatment for shock; summon help/transport to hospital; CPR, if necessary

23. antihistamine drugs for early signs and symptoms; glucocorticoids for severe or prolonged reactions
24. Latex sensitivity may result from a type I or type IV reaction. Type IV is the most common reaction, with a rash developing 48 to 96 hours after contact. Type I is rare but more serious, with possible asthma, hives, or anaphylaxis.

AUTOIMMUNITY

25. (Fig. 7.9) when individuals develop antibodies to their own cells or cellular material
26. Systemic lupus erythematosus (SLE) is diagnosed by the presence of numerous antinuclear antibodies (ANAs), especially anti-DNA, as well as other antibodies. Lupus erythematous (LE) cells are mature neutrophils containing nuclear material found in the circulating blood and are a positive sign.
27. prednisone (glucocorticoid) to reduce the immune response and subsequent inflammation; hydroxychloroquine (antimalarial) may be used to reduce exacerbations; nonsteroidal antiinflammatory drugs
28. (Table 7.7)
    i. skin: butterfly rash
    ii. joints: polyarthritis
    iii. heart: carditis and pericarditis
    iv. blood vessels: Raynaud's phenomenon
    v. blood: anemia, leukopenia, thrombocytopenia
    vi. kidneys: glomerulonephritis, with marked proteinuria and progressive damage
    vii. lungs: pleurisy
    viii. central nervous system: psychosis, depression, mood changes, seizures

IMMUNODEFICIENCY

29. (Table 7.8) primary: hypogammaglobulinemia; thymic aplasia, DiGeorge syndrome, combined immunodeficiency syndrome (CIDS), inherited deficits in any one or more of the components secondary: kidney disease, Hodgkin's disease, AIDS, radiation, immunosuppressive drugs, immunosuppression, malnutrition, loss or removal of the spleen, liver disease
30. predisposition to opportunistic infections and an increased risk of cancer
31. prophylactic antimicrobials to reduce incidence of opportunistic infections; gamma globulin replacement therapy to provide passive immunity (antibodies)

HIV AND AIDS

32. Human immunodeficiency virus (HIV) is the causative agent for AIDS. It is a "slow-acting" retrovirus containing two strands of RNA and the enzyme reverse transcriptase. Its envelope is characterized by spikes of glycoprotein. The virus is inactivated by many disinfectants and high temperatures.
33. CD4 T-helper lymphocytes are the major target and, when destroyed, their function in the initiation of both humoral and cellular immunity is reduced or absent.
34. HIV must enter the bloodstream of the recipient through transmission of body fluids such as blood, semen, and vaginal secretions. Transmission most often occurs through unprotected sexual intercourse with an HIV-positive partner, intravenous injection with contaminated needles, maternal-fetal transmission, or blood transfusion.
35. At the highest risk are intravenous drug users, people with multiple sexual partners (particularly those having unprotected sex), and the unborn fetuses of HIV-positive mothers.
36. (see also Figs. 7.13 and 7.14) Infected individuals usually become HIV positive within 2 to 10 weeks, but the "window" may be as long as 6 months. Full-blown AIDS may not occur for many years. After an initial infection, mild "flulike" symptoms appear in 3 to 6 weeks, followed by an asymptomatic latent period that may last for years before phase 3, acute onset of signs and symptoms, including multiple severe opportunistic infections and rare cancers such as Kaposi sarcoma.

Copyright © 2027 by Elsevier, Inc. All rights are reserved, including those for text and data mining, AI training, and similar technologies.

37. A blood test is performed for HIV antibodies using HIV antigen from recombinant HIV or ELISA for the primary test. The 3 stage process involves determining: 1. Presence of HIV-1/2 antigens/antibodies, differentiation/identification between HIV-1 and HIV-2 antibodies and a nucleic acid test to confirm HIV-1 positive and eliminate a false negative.
38. (Figs. 7.12 and 7.13) Full-blown AIDS may not occur for 6 to 7 years on average.
39. AIDS is diagnosed by a major decrease in the CD4 T-helper lymphocyte count and a change in the CD4+-to-CD8+ ratio in the presence of opportunistic infection or certain cancers.
40. (Fig. 7.13) mild, self-limited nonspecific "flulike" symptoms: low fever, fatigue, joint pain, and sore throat
41. (Fig. 7.15)
    i. generalized effects: lymphadenopathy, fatigue and weakness, headache, and arthralgia
    ii. opportunistic infections (see also gastrointestinal manifestations): *Pneumocystis carinii* in the lungs, causing severe pneumonia; herpes simplex, causing cold sores; and *Candida,* a fungus infection of the mouth and esophagus
    iii. gastrointestinal manifestations, including parasitical infections: chronic severe diarrhea, vomiting, and ulcers; necrotizing periodontal disease; severe weight loss, malnutrition, and wasting
    iv. oral manifestations: cold sores (herpes simplex) and *Candida*
    v. respiratory manifestations: *Pneumocystis carinii,* causing pneumonia
    vi. nervous system manifestations: HIV encephalopathy (AIDS dementia), aggravated by lymphomas, causing confusion, progressive cognitive impairment, memory loss, loss of coordination and balance, and depression; seizures
    vii. malignancies: Kaposi sarcoma and non-Hodgkin lymphomas
42. HIV drugs are grouped into six classes according to how they fight against HIV:
    - Nonnucleoside reverse transcriptase inhibitors (NNRTIs)
    - Nucleoside reverse transcriptase inhibitors (NRTIs)
    - Protease inhibitors (PIs)
    - Fusion inhibitors
    - CCR5 antagonists (CCR5s) (also called entry inhibitors)
    - Integrase strand transfer inhibitors (INSTIs)

    Antiviral drugs such as AZT; protease inhibitors such as indinavir; viral integrase inhibitors such as saquinavir and ritonavir; reverse transcriptase inhibitors such as zidovudine and lamivudine; and various drug combinations known as "cocktails", which can be made of combinations of 3 to 5 drugs; a "one pill daily" combination of three drugs (Atripla) is available to improve patient adherence to their drug protocol. Currently highly active antiretroviral (HAART) therapy has been very effective at controlling the virus, reducing the viral load in the blood, and returning CD4 cell counts to near-normal levels; prophylactic medications, including antibacterial, antifungal, and antituberculosis drugs; other drugs such as antidiarrheals (e.g., Imodium) and vitamin and mineral supplements may be required.
43. Prognosis is much improved because of earlier detection and newer drug and nutritional therapies. Without treatment, death occurs within several years of diagnosis.

CHAPTER 8: Skin Disorders

1. provides the first line of defense against invasion by microorganisms and other foreign material; prevents excessive fluid loss, important in controlling body temperature; provides sensory perception; synthesis and activation of vitamin D
2. See Fig. 8.1 of text.
    A. Hair, B. Capillaries, C. Sebaceous gland, D. Smooth muscle, E. Vein, F. Artery, G. Nerve fiber, H. Hair follicle, I. Adipose tissue, J. Subcutaneous tissue, K. Eccrine gland, L. Sensory receptor, M. Dermis, N. Stratum basale, O. Epidermis, P. Stratum corneum, Q. Melanocyte
3. They produce melanin, which protects the skin by absorbing and dispersing ultraviolet (UV) radiation, reducing DNA damage and lowering the risk of skin cancer.
4. Sebaceous glands produce sebum, an acidic oily secretion that inhibits bacterial growth, keeps the skin and hair soft, and reduces fluid loss. Eccrine glands secrete sweat through pores in response to heat or emotional stress.
5.

Condition	Etiology	Treatment
Scleroderma	Unknown; may be local or systemic	NSAIDs and glucocorticoids
Kaposi sarcoma	Rare skin cancer that occurs in immunosuppressed patients (especially patients with AIDS)	Radiation and chemotherapy
Tinea	Fungal infections of various parts of the body caused by various species of *Trichophyton*	Oral antifungal agents such as griseofulvin Topical antifungal agents: griseofulvin, tolnaftate, or ketoconazole
Atopic dermatitis	Type 1 hypersensitivity, with inherited tendency or genetic component	Topical glucocorticoids

Copyright © 2027 by Elsevier, Inc. All rights are reserved,
including those for text and data mining, AI training, and similar technologies.

Condition	Etiology	Treatment
Pemphigus	Autoimmune disorder	Systemic glucocorticoids
Herpes zoster	Varicella zoster virus	Antiviral medications for symptoms (e.g., acyclovir)
Herpes simplex	HSV-1	Topical acyclovir
Verrucae	Human papillomaviruses	Topical medications; laser and cryotherapy
Urticaria	Type 1 hypersensitivity to certain ingested substances (e.g., shellfish)	Topical antihistamines or topical glucocorticoids
Psoriasis	Unknown; familial tendency	Glucocorticoids; tar preparations, and methotrexate when severe
Scabies	Mite infection by *Sarcoptes scabiei*	Topical treatment with lindane
Lichen planus	Unknown inflammatory condition of skin and mucous membranes	Topical glucocorticoids
Impetigo	*Staphylococcus aureus*	Topical and systemic antimicrobials
Cellulitis	Infection of dermis and subcutaneous tissue, secondary to an injury; *S. aureus*	Systemic antimicrobials; local compression and analgesics
Necrotizing fasciitis	Group A β-hemolytic *Streptococcus*	Antimicrobials, fluid replacement, excision of all infected tissue, and amputation if necessary

6.
   i. those with excessive, cumulative sun (UV) exposure, smokers, people with scar tissue (particularly African Americans)
   ii. genetic predisposition; hormonal factors; UV radiation (sunlight)
   iii. immunosuppressed patients (e.g., people with AIDS)
7. a sore that does not heal; change in the shape, size, color, or texture of a lesion; new moles or the development of odd-shaped lesions; a skin lesion that bleeds repeatedly, oozes fluid, or itches
8. Diagnostic tests for skin lesions include culture and staining for bacterial infections, skin scrapings with microscopic examination, Wood's lamp evaluation for fungal infections, or parasitic infections. Biopsy (excisional, shave, or punch) is used to detect malignant changes. Blood tests, patch or scratch tests, and antigen–antibody testing help diagnose allergic or immune-related conditions.
9. See Fig. 8.2 of the text.
   A. Macule, B. Nodule, C. Papule, D. Pustule, E. Vesicle, F. Plaque, G. Ulcer, H. Fissure

CONSOLIDATION

10.
   i. Kaposi sarcoma
   ii. urticaria
   iii. pemphigus
   iv. scabies
   v. herpes simplex 1
   vi. verrucae
   vii. mycoses
   viii. atopic dermatitis
   ix. Dupuytren's contracture

11.
   1. Reducing sun exposure at midday and early afternoon
   2. Covering up with protective clothing or hats and staying in the shade
   3. Applying sunscreen to protect against UVA and UVB rays

CHAPTER 9: Musculoskeletal Disorders

FRACTURES

1. See Fig. 9.1*B* of the text.
   A. Articular cartilage, B. Epiphyseal line, C. Spongy bone, D. Compact bone, E. Medullary cavity, F. Nutrient foramen, G. Endosteum, H. Periosteum, I. Articular cartilage, J. Epiphysis, K. Diaphysis, L. Epiphysis
2. (Fig. 9.4)
   i. C: when the skin is broken; more damage to soft tissue (Open)
   ii. B: multiple fracture lines and bone fragments (Comminuted)
   iii. L: when a bone is crushed or collapses into small pieces (Compression)
   iv. H: bone is only partially broken, shaft is bent, tearing the cortical bone on one side (Greenstick)
   v. I: one end of the bone is forced or telescoped into the adjacent bone (Impacted)
   vi. A: fracture at an angle to the diaphysis of the bone (Oblique)
   vii. D: fracture results from a weakness in bone structure; due to tumor or osteoporosis (Pathological)
   viii. F: a break that angles around the bone; usually due to a twisting injury (Spiral)

Copyright © 2027 by Elsevier, Inc. All rights are reserved, including those for text and data mining, AI training, and similar technologies.

ix. G: a fracture across the bone (Transverse)
x. J: break in the distal radius at the wrist (Colles)
xi. E: a break in which several large bone fragments separate from the main body of a fractured bone
xii. K: fracture of the lower fibula at the ankle (Pott fracture)

3. (Fig. 9.5) Bleeding occurs and inflammation develops around the bone as a result of the soft tissue damage. A hematoma or clot forms in the medullary canal, under the periosteum. Necrosis occurs at the ends of the broken bone. The hematoma serves as a basis for fibrin network into which granulation tissue grows. Capillaries extend into tissue; phagocytic cells clean up debris. Fibroblasts (collagen) and chondroblasts (cartilage) migrate to the fibrin network. Bone ends become splinted by a procallus or fibrocartilaginous collar. Osteoblasts generate new bone, and callus is replaced, forming a bony callus. New bone is remodeled by osteoblastic and osteoclastic activity.
4. Complications include muscle spasm causing abnormalities in the bone during the healing process, infections, ischemia, compartment syndrome, fat emboli, nerve damage, nonunion (failure to heal) or malunion (deformity), and residual effects of fractures near a joint (osteoarthritis); stunted growth in children.
5. Reduction of a fracture is the manipulation of the fracture to restore bones to their normal position and alignment. A closed reduction is done by exerting pressure and traction. An open reduction requires surgery; devices may be placed to fix the fragments.
6. (Fig. 9.6) Dislocation is the separation of two bones at a joint with loss of contact between the articular surfaces. Subluxation is the partial displacement of bone with partial loss of contact between surfaces.
7. A sprain is a tear in a ligament. An avulsion occurs when a tendon or ligament is completely separated from its bony attachment.

BONE DISEASE

8. Diagnostic tools include: x-rays, CT scans, PET scans, and biopsy.
9.
   - aging
   - decreased mobility or sedentary lifestyle
   - hormonal factors such as hyperparathyroidism, Cushing's syndrome
   - deficits of calcium, vitamin D, or history of childhood deficits or malabsorption disorders
   - cigarette smoking
   - small, light bone structure
   - excessive caffeine intake
10. bones consisting of higher proportions of cancellous bone, such as vertebrae and the femoral neck
11. Osteopenia occurs as the bone density slowly becomes lower and is considered a midpoint on the progression to osteoporosis.
12. Bone resorption exceeds bone formation during the continuous process of bone remodeling, leading to thin, fragile bones.
13. Treatment includes dietary supplements, fluoride supplements, bisphosphonates, calcitonin, and human parathyroid hormone, weight-bearing exercises, raloxifene, and possibly newer medications under investigation such as strontium ranelate; antibody that binds to osteoclasts.
14.

	Rickets	**Osteomalacia**	**Paget Disease**
Etiology	Vitamin D deficiency in children due to diet or malabsorption	Vitamin D or calcium deficiency in adults	Idiopathic Unknown virus Genetic factors
Manifestations	Deformities—"bow legs" Decreased height	Soft bones Compression fractures	Pathological fractures Compression fractures of vertebrae; kyphosis Compression of cranial nerves Cardiovascular disease and heart failure
Treatment	Supplements Treat malabsorption	Supplements	Supportive

15. long-term use of phenobarbital (e.g., in treatment of seizures)
16. Osteosarcoma is a primary malignant neoplasm that usually develops in the metaphysis of the femur, tibia, or fibula in children or young adults, particularly males (Fig. 9.8). Chondrosarcomas are malignant tumors arising from cartilage and are more common in adults.

MUSCULAR DYSTROPHY

17. The basic pathophysiology is the same in all types of muscular dystrophy. A metabolic defect, a deficit of dystrophin, a muscle cell membrane protein, leads to degeneration and necrosis of the cell. Skeletal muscle fibers are replaced by fat and fibrous connective tissue, leading to the hypertrophic appearance of the muscle.
18. See Table 9.1.

Copyright © 2027 by Elsevier, Inc. All rights reserved,
including those for text and data mining, AI training, and similar technologies.

PRIMARILY FIBROMYALGIA SYNDROME

19. pain and stiffness affecting muscles, tendons, and surrounding soft tissues (not joints); other manifestations: sleep disturbances, depression, possibly irritable bowel syndrome, urinary symptoms

ARTHRITIS

20. It is a degenerative process. There is an increased incidence with age and excessive mechanical stress such as sports injuries or repetitive strain injury (RSI).
21. diagnosed by exclusion of other disorders and radiographic evidence of joint changes consistent with the clinical signs
22. (Figs. 9.10 to 9.14)

	Osteoarthritis	Rheumatoid Arthritis
Etiology	Degenerative Primary: idiopathic Secondary: injury Genetic factor	Autoimmune Genetic factor
Predisposing factors	Age Obesity Any joint injury Familial tendency	Familial predisposition Females
Joints involved	Weight-bearing and those frequently injured—hips and knees, cervical and lumbar spine, distal interphalangeal, temporomandibular	Symmetrical involvement Small joints of hands and feet Wrists and ankles Temporomandibular
Pathophysiology	Damage of articular cartilage leads to interference with movement, resulting in further damage, exposure of endochondral bone and development of cysts and osteophytes that causes joint space narrowing Inflammation in surrounding soft tissue	Synovitis leads to pannus formation, resulting in cartilage erosion, fibrosis, and finally ankylosis Muscle atrophy Development of malalignments, contractures, and deformities
Signs and symptoms	Pain with use Limited movement Enlarged, hard joints Crepitus No systematic manifestations	Aching and stiffness Impaired mobility Deformities, functional losses
Systemic effects	None	Rheumatoid factor (RF) in blood Elevated ESR Low-grade fever, malaise, fatigue Subcutaneous nodules: pleura, heart valves, eyes
Treatment	NSAIDs Minimize stress on joint Ambulatory aids Orthotic devices Arthroplasty Joint replacement	Physiotherapy; ambulatory aids Occupational therapy: assistive devices NSAIDs, COX-2 inhibitors Glucocorticoids Immunosuppressants Gold salts Arthroplasty Joint replacement

23.
- NSAIDs, COX-2 inhibitors
- glucocorticoids
- immunosuppressants
- gold salts
- Beta cell–depleting agents (rituximab)
- Interleukin-1 antagonists (anakinra)
- JAK Inhibitors (Janus Kinase)

24. The onset is usually more acute. Systemic effects are more marked, but rheumatoid nodules are absent. Large joints are frequently affected. Rheumatoid factor is not usually present. Other abnormal antibodies

Copyright © 2027 by Elsevier, Inc. All rights are reserved, including those for text and data mining, AI training, and similar technologies.

(e.g., ANA) may be present. The systemic form, Still's disease, develops with fever, rash, lymphadenopathy, and hepatomegaly, as well as joint involvement.

25. scaly skin patches, which may get worse when joint pain flares up, and flaky scalp
26. (Fig. 9.15) deposits of uric acid and urate crystals in the joint that cause an acute inflammatory response
27. Gout is usually due to a metabolic abnormality, resulting in hyperuricemia. It often affects only a single joint. It is more common in men older than age 40. There are tophi formation and urate crystal deposits.
28. Pathological changes include inflammation of the vertebral joints, fibrosis, and calcification or fusion of the joints, inflammation that begins in the lower back at sacroiliac joints and progresses up the spine, kyphosis, and osteoporosis; lung expansion may be limited at the late stage due to calcification of the costovertebral joints.

CONSOLIDATION

29.

i. osteoarthritis, rheumatoid arthritis
ii. gout
iii. rheumatoid arthritis
iv. rheumatoid arthritis
v. rheumatoid arthritis, gout, ankylosing spondylitis
vi. Duchenne's muscular dystrophy
vii. osteoporosis
viii. osteoarthritis
ix. fibromyalgia
x. rheumatoid arthritis
xi. rheumatoid arthritis
xii. osteoporosis, ankylosing spondylitis
xiii. rheumatoid arthritis, ankylosing spondylitis
xiv. rheumatoid arthritis
xv. gout
xvi. rheumatoid arthritis, ankylosing spondylitis
xvii. osteoarthritis, rheumatoid arthritis, gout, ankylosing spondylitis
xviii. rheumatoid arthritis
xix. osteoarthritis
xx. ankylosing spondylitis
xxi. osteoporosis
xxii. osteoarthritis
xxiii. osteoporosis
xxiv. myositis

CHAPTER 10: Blood and Circulatory System Disorders

ERYTHROCYTES

1. (Fig. 10.5 and 10.7) All blood cells originate in the red bone marrow from pluripotential hematopoietic stem cells during hemopoiesis. The life span is approximately 120 days. As the cell ages, it becomes rigid and fragile and finally is phagocytosed in the spleen or liver and broken down into globin and heme. Globin is broken down into amino acids and, along with the iron, is recycled to the liver to be used in hemoglobin synthesis. The heme is processed to release iron for recycling, and bilirubin, which is transported to the liver, where it is conjugated with glucuronide and then excreted in the bile.
2. (Handy Tables [inside back cover])
males: RBC: 4.9 to 5.9 × 106/mm^3 (4.9–5.9 × 1012/L)
hemoglobin: 13.5 to 18 g/100 mL (135–180 g/L)
females: RBC: 4.2 to 5.2 × 106/mm^3 (4.2–5.2 × 1012/L)
hemoglobin: 12 to 16 g/100 mL (120–160 g/L)
3. below normal concentrations of red blood cells and hemoglobin in the blood
4. fatigue, pallor, dyspnea, and tachycardia
5. (Table 10.2)

Type of Anemia	Etiology	Specific Signs and Symptoms	Specific Treatment
Iron deficiency anemia (Fig. 10.13)	Malnutrition Chronic blood loss Malabsorption Severe liver disease Underutilization of iron in some infections and cancers	Pallor Fatigue, lethargy, and cold intolerance Irritability Degenerative changes (e.g., brittle hair, rigid nails) Stomatitis and glossitis Menstrual irregularities Delayed healing Tachycardia, heart palpitations, dyspnea, and possible syncope	Identify and treat the underlying cause Iron supplements
Pernicious anemia—Vitamin B_{12} deficiency anemia (Fig. 10.14)	Dietary insufficiency (rare) Malabsorption resulting from autoimmune reaction; chronic gastritis; or inflammatory conditions (e.g., regional ileitis)	Basic signs of anemia Enlarged, red, sore tongue Decreased gastric acid leading to discomfort, nausea, and diarrhea Neurological effects: paresthesia in the extremities or loss of coordination and ataxia	Vitamin B_{12} injection

Copyright © 2027 by Elsevier, Inc. All rights are reserved, including those for text and data mining, AI training, and similar technologies.

Type of Anemia	Etiology	Specific Signs and Symptoms	Specific Treatment
Aplastic anemia	(Temporary or permanent) Idiopathic Myelotoxins (e.g., radiation, industrial chemicals, certain drugs)	Anemia (pallor, weakness, dyspnea) Leukopenia Thrombocytopenia (petechiae; excessive bleeding)	Prompt treatment of the underlying cause and removal of any bone marrow suppressants Blood transfusion Bone marrow transplant
Thalassemia	Genetic defect in which one or more genes for hemoglobin are missing or variant	Anemia (pallor, weakness, dyspnea)	Blood transfusion
Sickle cell anemia (Figs. 10.16, 10.17, 10.18)	Inherited characteristic leading to the formation of an abnormal hemoglobin (HbS)	Usually appears at about 1 year of age when fetal hemoglobin is replaced by HbS Severe anemia (pallor, weakness, tachycardia, and dyspnea) Hyperbilirubinemia (jaundice) Splenomegaly Painful crises due to vascular occlusion and infarction Delayed growth and development Congestive heart failure Frequent infections	Drugs that reduce sickling e.g., hydroxyurea) Avoidance of strenuous activity or high altitudes Supportive measures, including relief of pain

6. (Fig. 10.18) Inheritance pattern is autosomal recessive; the genotype of an individual with sickle cell anemia is homozygous.
7. The individual is heterozygous for sickle cell anemia. Less than half of his hemoglobin is abnormal; therefore, he experiences manifestations only in extreme circumstances.
8.
   i. 50%
   ii. 50%
   iii. 0%
   iv. 50%

	Mother With Sickle Cell Trait	
Father With Sickle Cell Anemia	HBs	HBa
HBss	HBss anemia	HBsa trait
HBss	HBss anemia	HBsa trait

9. (Fig. 10.17) An inherited, abnormal form of hemoglobin (HbS) is circulating in the bloodstream. When these RBCs are deoxygenated, they crystalize and change shape. The cell membrane is damaged, leading to hemolysis and shorter cell life span. The sickled cells cause vascular obstruction, thrombus formation, tissue infarction, and necrosis. Continued hemolysis results in severe anemia, hyperbilirubinemia, jaundice, splenomegaly, and gallstones.
10. (Figs. 10.10 and 10.17) deoxygenation of abnormal hemoglobin when O_2 levels are low
11. episodes caused by vascular occlusions and infarctions leading to permanent damage to organs and tissues; potential complications such as infection and congestive heart failure
12. (Fig. 10.17)
    i. excessive hemolysis, RBC breakdown, and resulting hyperbilirubinemia
    ii. cerebrovascular occlusion by sickled cells
    iii. diminished immune capacity (damage to spleen); vascular occlusions in the lungs; tissue damage and necrosis
    iv. congestion of the spleen due to presence of sickled cells in young people
    v. chronic stress on the heart due to efforts to improve oxygen supply and peripheral vascular resistance due to obstructions
13. genetic screening to identify carriers and genetic counseling to discern the risks of having a child with sickle cell anemia
14. Polycythemia is increased red blood cell and other cell production in the bone marrow.
15. Primary polycythemia is a neoplastic disorder of unknown origin, whereas secondary polycythemia may be a compensatory mechanism to provide increased oxygen transport in the presence of lung or heart disease or in people living at high altitudes.
16. *Signs and symptoms:* plethoric and cyanotic appearance; hepatomegaly; high blood pressure; full and bounding pulse; dyspnea, headaches, and visual disturbances. *Complications:* thromboses and infarctions in extremities, liver, kidneys, brain, and heart; congestive heart failure
17. immunosuppressive drugs, radiation, and periodic phlebotomy

Copyright © 2027 by Elsevier, Inc. All rights are reserved, including those for text and data mining, AI training, and similar technologies.

BLOOD CLOTTING

18. See Fig. 10.9 of the main text.
19. (Warning Signs of Excessive Bleeding Box) persistent bleeding from the gums or frequent nosebleeds, petechiae, frequent purpura and ecchymoses, abnormal persistent bleeding following trauma, bleeding into a joint, hemoptysis, hematemesis—vomiting blood, blood in the feces, anemia, feeling faint and anxious, low blood pressure, rapid pulse
20. CBC; hematocrit; hemoglobin; reticulocyte count; bone marrow aspiration and biopsy; serum iron, vitamin B_{12}, folic acid, cholesterol, urea, and bilirubin; bleeding time; prothrombin time; partial thromboplastin time
21. (Fig. 10.9) thrombocytopenia (many causes; e.g., autoimmune reactions): reduced circulating platelets that initiate the clotting process, defective platelet adhesion caused by ASA and NSAIDs, vitamin K deficiency: decreases prothrombin and fibrinogen levels liver disease: interferes with the production of clotting factors, inherited defects: cause deficiency in clotting factors, anticoagulant drugs (e.g., warfarin blocks prothrombin synthesis)
22. (Fig. 10.9)
    i. delayed clotting—due to decreased synthesis of clotting factors
    ii. delayed clotting—decreased aggregation or clumping of platelets
    iii. delayed clotting—vitamin K, which is necessary for production of clotting factors, is synthesized by resident flora of large intestine; prolonged antibiotic therapy may disrupt or destroy flora
    iv. delayed clotting—heparin inhibits thrombin formation
    v. delayed clotting—vitamin K necessary for synthesis of clotting factors by liver
    vi. promotes clotting—decreased blood velocity, resulting in pooling of blood
    vii. promotes clotting—increased blood viscosity, which decreases blood velocity and promotes pooling
    viii. delayed clotting—decreased platelets slow formation of platelet plug
    ix. promotes clotting—increased blood viscosity with resultant decreased blood velocity
    x. delayed clotting—anticoagulant that decreases synthesis of various clotting factors, particularly prothrombin
23. (Fig. 10.20) Hemophilia A is transmitted as an X-linked recessive trait and therefore it manifests in men, but women are carriers. Males are heterozygous; females are homozygous.
24.

	Female Carrier	
Father	**X**	**Xh**
X	XX normal female (25%)	X Xh (25%)
Y	XY normal male (25%)	Xh Y (25%)

    i. 25%—male
    ii. 25%—female
    iii. 50%
    iv. 50%
    v. 50%

25. (Fig. 10.20*B*)
    i. heterozygous
    ii. heterozygous
    iii. 50%
    iv. 25%
    v. female

	Mother	
Father	**XH**	**Xh**
XH	XHXH	XHXh
Y	XHY	XhY

26. (Fig. 10.21) Disseminated intravascular coagulation (DIC) involves excessive bleeding and clotting. It is a complication of numerous primary problems that activate the clotting process. Clotting causes multiple thromboses and infarctions but also consumes the available clotting factors and platelets. This can lead to hemorrhage and eventually hypotension or shock. Manifestations depend on the underlying cause. Hemorrhage is the most common critical problem combined with low blood pressure and possibly shock. Multiple bleeding sites are common, petechiae or ecchymoses may be present, mucosal bleeding is common, and hematuria may develop. Vascular occlusions may be present in the blood vessels. Difficulty in breathing and cyanosis are evident. Neurological effects include seizures and decreased responsiveness. Acute renal failure may accompany shock.

LEUKOCYTES

27. Leukemia is a neoplastic disorder involving one or more types of leukocytes that are present as undifferentiated, immature, nonfunctional cells that multiply uncontrollably and are found circulating in large numbers in the blood.
28. Blast cells are primitive undifferentiated nonfunctional stem cells seen in people with severe forms of acute leukemia.
29. (Table 10.3) acute or chronic; specific cell type involved: e.g., acute lymphocytic leukemia (ALL); chronic myelogenous leukemia (CML), etc.

Copyright © 2027 by Elsevier, Inc. All rights are reserved, including those for text and data mining, AI training, and similar technologies.

30. individuals with chromosomal abnormalities, particularly translocations such as Down syndrome; those exposed to radiation and certain chemicals

31. bone marrow biopsy

32.

Signs and Symptoms	Rationale
Weight loss and fatigue	Hypermetabolism associated with neoplastic growth, anorexia due to infection; pain; side effects of chemotherapy
Anemia	Due to hemorrhage and suppression of normal RBC production in the bone marrow
Thrombocytopenia	Suppression of platelet production in the bone marrow by proliferating neoplastic cells
Multiple infections, including those caused by microorganisms of low virulence	Nonfunctional WBCs being produced; diminished primary and secondary defense against infection
Increased bleeding and even severe hemorrhage	Thrombocytopenia
Kidney stones	Rapid turnover of cells leading to hyperuricemia
Fever	Hypermetabolism and/or infection
Lymphadenopathy	Excess production of abnormal leukocytes causes enlargement and congestion of lymphoid tissue
Splenomegaly and hepatomegaly	Excess production of abnormal leukocytes causes enlargement and congestion
Bone pain	Excessive cell production in the marrow causes pain due to pressure on nerves

33. (see Chapter 20) Chemotherapy, singly or in combinations, is the primary treatment. Adverse effects include bone marrow depression, nausea and vomiting, hair loss, and skin breakdown; some drugs cause pulmonary fibrosis. If ineffective, bone marrow transplantation is another intervention. Biological agents, such as interferon to stimulate the immune system, may also be used.

34. The best prognosis is in ALL in children between 1 and 9 years of age; less so in adolescents. The prognosis is poor in adults, especially those with AML. Patients with chronic leukemia may live up to 10 years. Prognosis depends on WBC and blast counts at diagnosis.

35.

	Acute Leukemia	Chronic Leukemia
Age of onset	Childhood and young adults	Older individuals
Course of disease	Acute onset; rapid development of manifestations	Insidious onset, milder, slower progression
Severity of symptoms	Acute	Milder
Number of blast cells	High	Fewer
Response to treatment	Very good in some types	Depends on general health

ATHEROSCLEROSIS

36. dietary modification; exercise program; cessation of smoking; drug therapy

37.

i. age—cannot be changed
ii. gender—cannot be changed
iii. genetic or familial factors—cannot be changed
iv. obesity—modifiable
v. cigarette smoking—modifiable
vi. sedentary lifestyle—modifiable
vii. diabetes mellitus—modifiable
viii. poorly controlled hypertension—modifiable

Copyright © 2027 by Elsevier, Inc. All rights are reserved, including those for text and data mining, AI training, and similar technologies.

ix. oral contraceptives and smoking in combination—modifiable
x. high cholesterol and hypertension—modifiable

38. (Fig. 10.26)
    i. Endothelial injury happens in the artery, often at a young age.
    ii. Inflammation and elevation of C-reactive protein develop.
    iii. White blood cells, especially monocytes and macrophages, accumulate.
    iv. Lipid accumulates in the intima or inner lining of the artery and media or muscle layer.
    v. A plaque forms and inflammation persists.
    vi. Platelets adhere to damaged surface, forming a thrombus and partial obstruction.
    vii. Lipid continues to build up at the site of injury, along with fibrous tissue (atheroma).
    viii. Platelets adhere, prostaglandins release, causing further inflammation and vasospasm.
    ix. Process continues with larger thrombus formation, potential for total occlusion, and possibility of embolism.
39. (Figs. 10.26 and 10.27) Development of atheromatous plaques narrows the lumen of arteries restricting flow, causing turbulence, thrombus formation, and potential embolism. The atheroma also damages the arterial wall, weakening the structure and decreasing elasticity, and ultimately may calcify, causing further rigidity. Complications include: 1) thrombus formation, with partial (angina); 2) total occlusion, precipitating a myocardial infarction; 3) embolism and infarction (stroke and peripheral vascular damage); 4) aneurysm; or 5) rupture and hemorrhage.
40. primarily large arteries particularly at bifurcations—aorta, coronary, iliac, carotids
41.
    i. Maintain weight at healthy levels to reduce the risk of metabolic syndrome, hypertension, and atherosclerosis.
    ii. Lower serum cholesterol and LDL in diet by reducing the intake of saturated fats and using unsaturated or vegetable oils; high dietary fiber intake also decreases LDL.
    iii. Minimize sodium intake to control hypertension.
    iv. Control primary disorders such as diabetes and hypertension.
    v. Cease smoking.
    vi. Exercise appropriate for age and health status to promote collateral circulation and reduce LDL levels.
    vii. Oral anticoagulant therapy can be used in case of thrombus formation concern.
    viii. Surgical intervention may be necessary.
42. (Table 12.1)
    i. lower cholesterol and LDL levels
    ii. lower platelet aggregation, leading to a lower chance of thrombosis and thus leading to a lower chance of heart attacks and strokes
    iii. interfere with clotting factor synthesis (warfarin) or inhibit thrombin formation (heparin), leading to a lower chance of thrombosis and a lower chance of heart attacks and strokes
    iv. help decrease cardiac workload
43. percutaneous transluminal coronary angioplasty (PTCA); coronary artery bypass grafting (CABG); laser angioplasty
44. Signs include fatigue, weakness, and intermittent claudication (leg pain during exercise) that worsens over time. Symptoms also include paresthesias (tingling, numbness), weak/absent pulses, and skin changes like pallor, cyanosis, dryness, hairlessness, and thickened toenails.
45. Varicose veins result from dilated veins due to weak vein walls or defective valves, often in the legs. Weak walls stretch under pressure, and damaged valves cause blood backflow, increasing venous pressure, edema, and risks of ulcers or thrombosis.
46. Thrombophlebitis is vein inflammation causing thrombus formation with pain, swelling, and redness; phlebothrombosis is spontaneous, asymptomatic thrombus formation. Venous thrombosis can lead to pulmonary embolism, where a clot fragment blocks lung arteries, causing chest pain and shock.

CONSOLIDATION

47.
    i. disseminated intravascular coagulation (DIC)
    ii. pernicious anemia
    iii. leukemia (especially acute)
    iv. hemophilia A
    v. polycythemia
    vi. aplastic anemia, leukopenia, thrombocytopenia
    vii. sickle cell anemia
    viii. thalassemia
    ix. sickle cell anemia
    x. pernicious anemia, vitamin B_{12} deficiency anemia
    xi. polycythemia vera
    xii. leukemia
    xiii. leukemia, anemia (especially aplastic and sickle cell), Hodgkin's, multiple myeloma

CHAPTER 11: Lymphatic System Disorders

LYMPHATIC SYSTEM STRUCTURES

1. A. Tonsil, B. Left subclavian vein, C. Bone marrow, D. Spleen, E. Inguinal lymph nodes, F. Thoracic duct, G. Axillary lymph nodes, H. Thymus, I. Right subclavian vein, J. Right lymphatic duct, K. Lymph capillaries, L. Blood capillary, M. Tissue cells, N. Venule, O. Arteriole

LYMPHATIC SYSTEM DISORDERS

2. (Fig. 11.8) Giant Reed-Sternberg cell is used for diagnosis. It is characterized as a giant irregular cell present in the lymph node.

Copyright © 2027 by Elsevier, Inc. All rights are reserved, including those for text and data mining, AI training, and similar technologies.

3. (Fig. 11.9) stage I—single lymph node or region; stage II—multiple regions on same side of diaphragm; stage III—lymph node regions on both sides of diaphragm; stage IV—widespread; liver and spleen
4. large, painless, nontender lymph node, usually in the neck; splenomegaly and enlarged lymph nodes at other locations later; general signs of cancer such as weight loss, anemia, low-grade fever, night sweats, and fatigue; recurrent infection
5. Chemotherapy is the first preferred method. Radiation and surgery also prove effective. In advanced cases, stem cell transplants along with immune-chemotherapy can be used.
6. Non-Hodgkin lymphoma is distinguished by multiple node involvement scattered throughout the body in a nonorganized pattern of widespread metastasis; intestinal nodes are frequently involved in the early stages.
7. a neoplastic disease of unknown etiology involving plasma cells
8. Signs and symptoms include frequent infections due to impaired antibody production; bone pain due to production of excess plasma cells in the marrow; pathological fractures due to the weakened bones; anemia and bleeding tendencies because blood cell production is compromised; and proteinuria due to altered kidney function.
9. Although not always required, the following treatment methods are available: targeted chemotherapy, CAR (chimeric antigen receptor)-T-cell therapy, corticosteroids/analgesics, bone marrow transplants, radiation therapy.

CHAPTER 12: Cardiovascular System Disorders

HEART

1. See Figs. 12.1, 12.3, and 12.10.
   A. Left atrium, B. Left AV (mitral) valve, C. Left ventricle, D. Papillary muscle, E. Interventricular septum, F. Pericardium, G. Chordae tendineae, H. Interior vena cava, I. Right ventricle, J. Right AV (tricuspid) valve, K. Right atrium, L. Aortic semilunar valve, M. Superior vena cava, N. Aorta

ANGINA PECTORIS (AP)

2. chest pain
3.
   i. when there is decreased blood supply (oxygen) to the heart, due to either arterial obstruction or spasm OR
   ii. when there is increased demand for oxygen by the heart OR
   iii. when there is a combination of factors
4. a. atherosclerosis, b. arteriosclerosis, c. vasospasm, d. myocardial hypertrophy, e. severe anemias, f. respiratory disease
5. myocardial infarction
6. (answers throughout chapter)
   i. smoke causes vasoconstriction, leading to increased venous return and increased heart rate
   ii. vasoconstriction, leading to increased venous return and increased heart rate
   iii. sympathetic stimulation increases heart rate
   iv. increases heart rate due to increased O_2 demands
7. The classic manifestations are recurrent, intermittent brief episodes of substernal chest pain, described as a tightness or pressure that may radiate to the neck or left arm. An anginal attack usually lasts a few seconds or minutes.
8. Coronary vasodilators, such as nitroglycerin, act by reducing systemic resistance, thus decreasing the demand for oxygen. Some vasodilators also relieve arterial vasospasm. Nitroglycerin has an immediate onset of action.
9. sublingual
10. See Emergency Treatment for Angina Attack Box.
11. (Emergency Treatment for Angina Attack Box)
    i. if pain is not relieved with rest and administration of three doses of nitroglycerin spaced 5 minutes apart—*i.e.,* after 10 minutes
    ii. for individual with no history of angina, if pain is unrelieved within 2 minutes
12. (Table 12.1)

Drug Group	Action and Effects	Adverse Effects	Example
β-Adrenergic blockers	Blocks β-adrenergic receptors, slowing the heart rate, reducing work of the heart	Dizziness, fatigue	Metoprolol (Lopressor)
Calcium channel blockers	Vasodilator, blocks calcium channel, reducing cardiac contractility and work	Dizziness, fainting, headache	Nifedipine (Adalat)
Nitrates (vasodilators; transdermal or oral form)	Reduces cardiac workload; decreases peripheral resistance by vasodilation	Dizziness; headache	Nitroglycerin

i. antihypertensive to lower blood pressure and cardiac workload
ii. diuretic to help control blood pressure and prevent edema
iii. platelet inhibitor to lower platelet aggregation and the chance of thrombus formation

Copyright © 2027 by Elsevier, Inc. All rights are reserved, including those for text and data mining, AI training, and similar technologies.

iv. antihyperlidemic to lower blood cholesterol and LDL levels and hopefully slow or arrest progression of atherosclerosis

14. (Fig. 12.12) angioplasty and stent insertion; coronary bypass graft
15.
    i. Avoid situations known to precipitate attacks (e.g., stress).
    ii. Stop smoking.
    iii. Consume diet low in saturated and trans fats.
    iv. Restrict sodium intake.
    v. Lose weight if overweight.
    vi. Engage in a consistent exercise program.
    vii. Reduce stress.
16.
    i. How long has he had angina?
    ii. How frequent are the attacks?
    iii. When was the last one?
    iv. What are the known precipitating factors?
    v. What is his response to nitroglycerin?
    vi. Does he have his nitroglycerin with him?
    vii. Has he suffered a heart attack?
17.
    i. stress reduction—explanations and reassurance
    ii. prophylactic use of nitroglycerin

MYOCARDIAL INFARCTION

18. death of cardiac muscle resulting from prolonged ischemia
19. MIs are generally classified as either ST-elevation MIs (STEMI) or non-ST elevation MI (NSTEMI) based on specific characteristics of their ECGs. MIs are then further divided into five different types. Type 1 is primarily associated with atherosclerosis and the destruction of cardiac muscle due to blockage of a major artery/arteries. Type 2 is characterized by a mismatch in myocardial oxygen supply and demand that is not a direct result of arterial blockage. Type 3 involves only fatal Mis, and Types 4 and 5 are attributed to MIs that occur as a result of a medical procedure(s) such as angioplasty or stents.
20. Infarction may develop in three ways:
    i. thrombus buildup to obstruct the artery due to atherosclerosis (most common)
    ii. vasospasm in the presence of a partial occlusion
    iii. embolization of a thrombus to a smaller artery that is totally obstructed
21. pallor, anxiety, fear, diaphoresis, shortness of breath and tightness in chest, weakness, indigestion, or nausea
22. Transmural infarction involves all three layers of heart.
23. left ventricle
24. (Fig. 12.10) Myocardial infarction occurs when a coronary artery is totally occluded, causing prolonged ischemia and cell death or infarction of the myocardium. At the point of obstruction, heart tissue becomes necrotic, and an area of injury, inflammation, and ischemia develops around the necrotic zone. Functions of myocardial contractility and conduction are lost quickly. There is irreversible damage unless blood supply can be restored with the first 20 to 30 minutes. Inflammation subsides after 48 hours. The area of necrosis is gradually replaced by fibrous (nonfunctional) tissue. The size of the infarct is determined by location of arterial blockage and presence of collateral circulation.
25. Signs and symptoms include sudden, severe, steady, and crushing substernal chest pain that radiates to the left arm, shoulder, jaw, or neck. Other manifestations may occur even if pain is not present, including pallor, diaphoresis, nausea, dizziness, weakness, dyspnea, anxiety, fear, hypotension, and low-grade fever.
26. Diagnosis is confirmed through electrocardiogram (ECG) changes and serum enzyme and isoenzyme levels. Serum levels of myosin and cardiac troponin are elevated; serum electrolyte levels may be abnormal; leukocytosis and an elevated C-reactive protein (CRP) and erythrocyte sedimentation rate (ESR) are common; arterial blood gas is altered. Pulmonary artery pressure measurements should be conducted to determine ventricular function.
27. (Fig. 12.15) Serum enzymes are intracellular enzymes diffused from necrotic cells into the serum in a typical and predictable pattern that can be measured. Isoenzymes are subgroups of a specific enzyme and are found primarily in one type of tissue. Levels of serum enzymes and isoenzymes can be used to identify the site of the infarction, confirm a myocardial infarction, and assess size (severity) of infarction.
28. Electrical activity of myocardium will be altered in areas of severe ischemia or necrosis.
29. Arrhythmias account for the greatest number of deaths because they impair the efficiency of the heart, resulting in decreased perfusion to vital organs as well as the heart itself, leading to shock.
30. Other complications include cardiogenic shock, congestive heart failure, and, less frequently, the rupture of necrotic heart tissue and thromboembolism.
31. Treatment includes rest—which allows body to repair damage without stressors; oxygen therapy—which increases oxygen levels to compensate for decreased cardiac output; analgesics—which relieve pain; anticoagulants—to prevent clot formation; antiarrhythmic drugs—which reduce arrythmias; digoxin—which generally supports heart function; specific measure to treat shock if present—which reduce chances of another attack or development of congestive heart failure; and bypass surgery—which can redirect blood supply around damaged vessels.
32.
    i. Angina is usually precipitated by something that increases heart rate; a myocardial infarction (MI) may occur at rest or even while asleep.
    ii. Anginal pain is relieved by nitroglycerin and rest; the pain of an MI is not relieved by nitroglycerin and rest.
    iii. There is no tissue death (permanent damage) with angina; MI causes cell death.

Copyright © 2027 by Elsevier, Inc. All rights are reserved,
including those for text and data mining, AI training, and similar technologies.

iv. Cardiac enzymes and isoenzymes are elevated with MI; there are no changes with angina. There are permanent ECG changes with MI; no permanent ECG change occurs with angina.
v. There is leukocytosis with MI; white blood cell count is not elevated with angina.
vi. CRP is elevated with MI; it is not elevated with angina.
vii. ESR is elevated with MI but not with angina.
viii. There are elevated serum levels of myosin and troponin with MI.

CARDIAC DYSRHYTHMIAS (ARRHYTHMIAS)

33. (See Fig. 12.2)
34. (Fig. 12.2) SA node to AV node to AV bundle (bundle of His) to right and left bundle branches to Purkinje fibers
35. (See Fig. 12.2)
36.
    i. P wave: atrial depolarization
    ii. QRS complex: ventricular depolarization
    iii. T wave: ventricular repolarization
37. alteration of cardiac rate or rhythm
38. Cardiac arrhythmias may be due to damage to the heart's conduction system or to systemic causes such as electrolyte abnormalities, fever, hypoxia, stress, infection, or drug toxicity.
39. (Table 12.2)
    a) heart rate greater than 350 beats per minute; v. fibrillation
    b) extra heartbeat arising in the ventricles; viii. premature ventricular contraction (PVC)
    c) heart rate less than 60 beats per minute; ii. bradycardia
    d) slowing or no transmission of impulses between atria and ventricles; vi. heart block
    e) additional heartbeat originating in atria; vii. premature atrial contraction (PAC)
    f) restoration of normal cardiac rhythm by electrical shock; i. cardioversion
    g) heart rate between 160 and 350 beats per minute; iv. flutter
    h) extra beat originating outside the SA node; iii. ectopic beat
    i) heart rate between 100 and 160 beats per minute; ix. tachycardia
40. It interferes with normal ventricular filling and decreases both period of ventricular diastole and perfusion.
41. It results in decreased cardiac output, which results in decreased perfusion of vital organs.
42. (Table 12.1)

Drug Group	Action and Effects	Adverse Effects	Example
β-Adrenergic blockers	Blocks β-adrenergic receptors, slowing the heart rate, prevents sympathetic nervous system (SNS) stimulation and increased demand on heart	Dizziness, fatigue	Metoprolol (Lopressor)
Calcium channel blockers	Vasodilator, blocks calcium channel	Dizziness, fainting, headache	Nifedipine (Adalat)
Digitalis (cardiac glycosides)	Slows conduction through the atrioventricular (AV) node, increases force of contraction (cardiotonic) to increase efficiency	Nausea, fatigue, headache, weakness	Digoxin (Lanoxin)

43. (Table 12.1)
    - antihypertensive to decrease blood pressure and cardiac workload
    - diuretic to help control blood pressure and prevent edema
    - platelet inhibitor to decrease platelet aggregation and decrease the chance of thrombus formation
    - anticoagulant to decrease the chance of thrombus formation
    - antihyperlidemic to decrease blood cholesterol and LDL levels and hopefully slow or arrest progression of atherosclerosis
    - nitroglycerin
44. device that provides electrical stimulation directly to the heart muscle to stimulate heart contraction as needed or to gain overall control of heart rate
45. Use of electronic equipment (microwaves, dental Cavitrons) may interfere with normal functioning of pacemaker.

cessation of all activity in the heart—no impulse conduction, thus a flat ECG

HEART FAILURE

47. Causes include a problem in the heart itself (e.g., valve defect or MI) or a condition that increases the workload of the heart (e.g., hypertension).
48. (Fig. 12.16) Reduced blood flow into systemic circulation to include kidneys: increased rennin and aldosterone secretion—resulting in vasoconstriction and increased blood volume. SNS response increases heart rate and peripheral resistance. Chambers of the heart tend to dilate, and cardiac muscle becomes hypertrophied.
49. (Fig. 12.17) Backward effects: the chamber and blood vessels behind or "upstream" from the failing ventricle will not empty properly, resulting in the accumulation or congestion of blood and therefore an increased pressure in these areas. Forward effects: there will be decreased output of blood from the failing ventricle into the vessels "in front" of it or "downstream."

Copyright © 2027 by Elsevier, Inc. All rights are reserved, including those for text and data mining, AI training, and similar technologies.

50. (Table 12.3)

	Right-Sided Heart Failure	Left-Sided Heart Failure
Cause	Infarction of right ventricle, pulmonary valve stenosis, pulmonary disease (cor pulmonale)	Infarction of left ventricle, aortic valve stenosis, hypertension, hyperthyroidism
Backward effects	Dependent edema in feet, hepatomegaly and splenomegaly, ascites, distended neck veins, headache, flushed face	Orthopnea, cough, shortness of breath, paroxysmal nocturnal dyspnea, hemoptysis, rales
Forward effects	Fatigue, weakness, dyspnea, exercise intolerance, cold intolerance	Fatigue, weakness, dyspnea, exercise intolerance, cold intolerance
Manifestations	See above forward and backward effects. Compensations: tachycardia and pallor, secondary polycythemia, daytime oliguria	See above forward and backward effects. Compensations: tachycardia and pallor, secondary polycythemia, daytime oliguria

51.
- i. venous congestion in the inferior vena cava causes blood pooling in the spleen
- ii. venous congestion in the inferior vena cava causing fluid to shift into the peritoneal cavity
- iii. due to pulmonary edema—fluid shifts into upper lobes when head lowered, causing dyspnea and anxiety, and more fluid shifts from tissues into blood when recumbent, thus increasing vascular volume and pressure in pulmonary capillaries
- iv. due to fluid congestion in lungs and pulmonary edema
- v. as congestion increases in pulmonary circulation, red blood cells are pushed out of capillaries into alveoli, causing rusty-colored sputum or blood-specked sputum
- vi. due to increased congestion and pressure in superior vena cava
- vii. occurs during day—vas fluid accumulates in dependent regions, and there is decreased renal perfusion; late in disease, oliguria reflects decreased cardiac output and renal failure
- viii. when individual is in supine position, edema in dependent areas is mobilized, resulting in increased cardiac output, renal perfusion, and therefore glomerular filtration rate
- ix. impaired gas exchange due to pulmonary congestion causes chronic hypoxia that in turn stimulates release of erythropoietin—increased RBC production

52.
- i. helps prevent fluid retention
- ii. could help arrest progression of atherosclerosis
- iii. prevent venous stasis and thrombophlebitis
- iv. decreases dyspnea and improves arterial blood gases
- v. mobilize edema (including pulmonary edema) and promote excretion of excess fluid, leading to decreased plasma volume and therefore decreased cardiac workload
- vi. prevents hypokalemia, which is a common side effect of diuretic therapy
- vii. decrease renin secretion and therefore prevent both vasoconstriction and aldosterone secretion (which causes salt and water retention)
- viii. increases strength of myocardial contractions that increase cardiac output
- ix. decreases thrombosis, particularly in legs
- x. decreases anxiety, which can contribute to increased heart and respiratory rates

CONGENITAL HEART DEFECTS

53. Most defects are multifactorial and reflect both genetic and environmental influences (e.g., chromosomal abnormalities in Down syndrome). Environmental factors include viral infections such as rubella and maternal alcoholism (fetal alcohol syndrome [FAS]) and maternal diabetes.

54. (Fig. 12.20)
- i. a hole or defect in the atrial or ventricular septa
- ii. failure of a valve to close completely
- iii. backward flow or leaking of blood due to valvular incompetence
- iv. abnormally enlarged and floppy valve leaflets that balloon backward with pressure or posterior displacement of the valve cusp
- v. narrowing of a valve
- vi. abnormal heart sounds due to leaky valves

55. by presence of a heart murmur

56. Left-to-right shunt means that blood from the left side of the heart is recycled to the right side and to the lungs, resulting in increased volume in the pulmonary circulation, decreased cardiac output, and an inefficient system—an acyanotic condition. Right-to-left shunt means that unoxygenated blood from the right side of the heart bypasses the lung directly and enters the left side of the heart and hence the systemic circulation, producing varying degrees of cyanosis; death may occur in infancy in severe cases.

57. Signs and symptoms include:
- pallor and cyanosis
- tachycardia, with very rapid sleeping pulse, frequently a pulse deficit
- dyspnea on exertion and tachypnea
- in toddlers and older children, frequently assuming a squatting position to modify blood flow
- clubbed fingers developed in time
- marked intolerance for exercise and exposure to cold
- delayed growth and development

Copyright © 2027 by Elsevier, Inc. All rights are reserved,
including those for text and data mining, AI training, and similar technologies.

58. Ventricular septal defect is the most common congenital heart defect—"hole in the heart." Large openings: left-to-right shunt, reducing the flow of blood from the left ventricle, reducing stroke volume and cardiac output in the systemic circulation. More blood enters the pulmonary circulation, compromising its efficiency, and in time, overloads and irreversibly damages the pulmonary vessels, causing pulmonary hypertension. This complication, if untreated, would lead to abnormally high pressure in the right ventricle and reversal of the shunt to a right-to-left shunt, leading to cyanosis.

59.

Defect	Backward Effects	Forward Effects	Manifestations
Mitral stenosis	Left atrial hypertrophy Atrial arrhythmias Mural thrombi Pulmonary congestion Pulmonary hypertension	Decreased cardiac output	Dyspnea, orthopnea Cyanosis, fatigue Arrhythmias Heart murmur Increased risk of stroke due to emboli originating in left atrium
Mitral regurgitation	Left atrial hypertrophy Atrial arrhythmias Mural thrombi Pulmonary congestion Pulmonary hypertension	Decreased cardiac output	Dyspnea, orthopnea Cyanosis, fatigue, dizziness Arrhythmias Heart murmur
Aortic stenosis	Left ventricular hypertrophy If severe, increased congestion in left atrium and pulmonary congestion	Decreased cardiac output	Dizziness, fainting Fatigue Heart murmur If severe, dyspnea, orthopnea, cyanosis, angina
Aortic regurgitation	Left ventricular hypertrophy If severe, heart failure	Increased stroke volume and cardiac output	Very strong, bounding pulse Heart murmur May develop symptoms of heart failure
Pulmonary stenosis	Right ventricular hypertrophy Congestion in right atrium and systemic veins Leads to right-sided heart failure	Decreased blood flow through pulmonary circulation, leading to decreased gas exchange and blood to left side of heart	Weakness, fatigue, cyanosis Swelling of feet and ankles Symptoms of right-sided heart failure Heart murmur
Pulmonary regurgitation	Right ventricular hypertrophy Congestion in right atrium and systemic veins Leads to right-sided heart failure	Decreased blood flow through pulmonary circulation, leading to decreased gas exchange and blood to left side of heart	Weakness, fatigue, cyanosis Swelling of feet and ankles Symptoms of right-sided heart failure Heart murmur

60. valvular defect; septal defect
61. (Fig. 12.25*E*)
   i. pulmonary valve stenosis: restricts outflow from the right ventricle, leading to right ventricular hypertrophy and high pressure in the right ventricle leading to the right-to-left shunt
   ii. ventricular septal defect (VSD): an opening in the ventricular septum allows blood to flow between the ventricles
   iii. dextroposition of the aorta: promotes blood flow directly from the right ventricle into the general circulation
   iv. right ventricular hypertrophy: thickening of the ventricular wall because of increased work

   The most common cyanotic congenital heart disorder, tetralogy of Fallot, is a right-to-left shunt of blood through the VSD with marked systemic effects. This means that unoxygenated blood from the right side of the heart bypasses the lungs and enters the left side of the heart and into the general circulation. The high proportion of unoxygenated blood produces a bluish color in the skin and mucous membranes (cyanosis) and marked systemic effects resulting from hypoxemia.
62. Treatments include surgical repair of defect, valve replacement, or drug therapy (those used for heart failure).
63.
   i. He will be taking a platelet inhibitor such as ASA or an anticoagulant because despite replacement of damaged valve, platelets will still aggregate on the replacement. These could become emboli, therefore increasing risk of stroke.

Copyright © 2027 by Elsevier, Inc. All rights are reserved, including those for text and data mining, AI training, and similar technologies.

ii. He will require an antibacterial agent, preferably penicillin (unless he is allergic) for prophylaxis, because invasive procedures provide a portal of entry for bacteria that may then colonize the prosthetic valve, causing infective endocarditis.

RHEUMATIC FEVER, RHEUMATIC HEART DISEASE, AND INFECTIVE ENDOCARDITIS

64. group A β-hemolytic streptococci
65. those between the age of 5 and 15 years
66. An acute systemic inflammatory condition resulting from abnormal immune reaction of an untreated infection, usually β streptococci. Results in acute cardiac inflammation involving one or more layers of the heart: pericarditis, myocarditis, and/or endocarditis. Other sites of inflammation include large joints, particularly in the legs; migratory polyarthritis; nonpruritic skin rash; nontender subcutaneous nodules on the extensor surfaces of wrists, elbows, knees, or ankles; and inflammation of the basal nuclei in the brain, causing involuntary jerky movements. Rheumatic heart disease can develop years later.
67.
    i. low-grade fever, leukocytosis, malaise, anorexia, and fatigue
    ii. inflammation of the outer layer of the heart; may include effusion
    iii. inflammation develops as localized lesions in the heart muscle, called Aschoff bodies
    iv. inflammation of the inner lining of the heart, especially the valves, which become edematous; verrucae (small wartlike lesions) form
    v. migratory inflammation of many joints, especially in the legs
    vi. erythema marginatum (red macules or papules)
    vii. nontender lesions on the extensor surfaces of wrists, elbows, and knees
    viii. inflammation of the basal nuclei in the brain causing involuntary jerky movements of the face, arms, and legs
68. Endocarditis may lead to permanent scarring of heart valves, which leads to rheumatic heart disease. If rheumatic heart disease develops, the individual is now at high risk for infective endocarditis.
69. CBC (Chapter 11) and serology for identifying leukocytosis and anemia; monitoring antistreptolysin O antibody titer; ECG to identify characteristic changes
70.

Medication	**Effects**	**Example**
Antibiotics	Eradicate bacteria and prevent further infection	Penicillin (first choice unless patient is allergic)
NSAIDs	Decrease acute inflammation to prevent heart complications Relieve joint symptoms Lower fever	ASA Ibuprofen
Corticosteroids	Decrease immune response and acute inflammation to prevent heart complications	Prednisone
Antipyretics	Decrease fever	ASA Ibuprofen Acetaminophen
Antiarrhythmics	Improve efficiency of heart function and prevent complications	Metoprolol Nifedipine Digoxin
Muscle relaxants	Decrease muscle spasms	Diazepam

71. restriction of physical activities; maintenance of nutrition and hydration
72. (Figs. 12.23 and 12.24) Rheumatic fever is an acute, inflammatory disorder caused by abnormal immune response, following an infection by group A β-hemolytic streptococci. Rheumatic heart disease is a long-term result of rheumatic fever that involves permanent scarring of one or more heart valves and a high risk of infective endocarditis. Scar tissue in the myocardium may cause arrhythmias.
73. mitral valve
74. Damaged heart valve stimulates platelet aggregation, leading to increased risk of emboli and stroke.
75. Damaged endocardial surface provides environment for bacterial colonization.
76. Some individuals should be premedicated with antimicrobial drugs before invasive procedures to avoid bacteremia. There are two predisposing factors for subacute infective endocarditis: damaged endocardium and portal of entry for bacteria or other organisms. Someone with rheumatic heart disease has

Copyright © 2027 by Elsevier, Inc. All rights are reserved,
including those for text and data mining, AI training, and similar technologies.

damaged heart valves, and the invasive procedure provides the portal of entry.

77. Despite replacement of damaged valve, there is an increased susceptibility to thrombus formation, requiring patients to take daily ASA (Fig. 12.26*B*).
78. subacute: defective heart valves infected by organisms with low virulence (i.e., *Streptococcus viridans*); acute: normal valves attacked by highly virulent pathogens (i.e., *Staphylococcus aureus*)
79. Those with:
    - congenital defects
    - rheumatic fever
    - mitral prolapse
    - prosthetic heart valve(s)
    - septal defects
    - recent stent insertion (artificial)
    - indwelling catheters
    - immunosuppression or immunodeficiency such as AIDS
80.
    - infection of normal or defective heart valves
    - inflammation of the valves and formation of vegetations on the cusps
    - defective opening and closing of valves
    - potential for septic emboli causing infarction or infection
    - additional scarring and destruction of valve leaflets and chordae tendinea
81. Subacute infective endocarditis has an insidious onset. Various new heart murmurs are common. An initial low-grade fever and fatigue may be signs. Anorexia, splenomegaly, and Osler's nodes on the fingers are often present. There are signs of vascular occlusion or infection (abscesses) in remote locations. An intermittent high fever (septicemia) may develop, and in severe cases, congestive heart failure develops. Acute endocarditis has a sudden onset with sudden spiked fever, chills, and drowsiness. Heart valves are badly damaged and may be torn, causing severe impairment of heart function. As in the subacute form, septic emboli may cause infarctions and abscesses in remote sites with corresponding signs and symptoms of infection.
82. blood culture
83. antimicrobial drugs, usually for a minimum of 4 weeks; other medication to support heart function is usually required
84.

	Rheumatic Fever	Infective Endocarditis
Causative agent(s)	Group A β-hemolytic streptococci	Acute *Staphylococcus aureus* (most common) Subacute *Streptococcus viridans* (most common) Gram-negative bacilli Enterococci Fungi
Predisposing factors	Age: 5–15 Economically disadvantaged Living in crowded conditions	Damaged endocardium: rheumatic heart disease, previous endocarditis, congenital heart defects, prosthetic heart valves Portal of entry for microbes: IV drug users, indwelling catheters, recent joint replacement
Manifestations and complications	General: fever, leukocytosis, malaise, fatigue, anorexia Heart: pericarditis, myocarditis, endocarditis, tachycardia, heart murmur, arrhythmias, heart failure Polyarthritis Skin manifestations: rash Chorea Subcutaneous nodules Epistaxis Abdominal pain	General: fever, leukocytosis, fatigue, anorexia, elevated ESR Positive blood culture Change in heart murmur Septic emboli Cough, dyspnea Arthralgia, arthritis Petechial hemorrhages in skin, mucosa, nail bed Chest pain Confusion, paralysis, stroke Blindness Hematuria Abdominal pain
Antibiotic of choice	Penicillin	Penicillin or other drug specific for causative agent
Prophylactic antibiotic coverage?	Not unless permanent heart valve problems (*i.e.,* rheumatic heart disease); then amoxicillin	Yes—amoxicillin unless allergic

'5. Acute pericarditis may involve a simple inflammation of the pericardium or may be secondary to open heart surgery, myocardial infarction, rheumatic fever, systemic lupus erythematosus, cancer, renal failure, trauma, or viral infection.

HYPERTENSION

86. High blood pressure, when the systolic pressure is above 120 and the diastolic pressure is above 70 when an individual is at rest. Essential hypertension develops

Copyright © 2027 by Elsevier, Inc. All rights reserved, including those for text and data mining, AI training, and similar technologies.

when blood pressure is consistently above 140/90 mm Hg. Men are more likely to have hypertension before age 55, after which age women have a greater incidence. Differences in systolic and diastolic pressure increase with age, as the elasticity of arteries is lost.

87. Essential hypertension is idiopathic. Secondary hypertension results from renal (e.g., nephrosclerosis) or endocrine (e.g., hyperaldosteronism) disease, or pheochromocytoma.
88. hypertension that is uncontrollable, severe, and rapidly progressive with many complications and characterized by high diastolic pressure
89.
    - genetic factors—nonmodifiable
    - excessive alcohol intake—modifiable
    - high sodium intake—modifiable
    - obesity—modifiable
    - prolonged or recurrent stress—modifiable
90. There is an increase in arteriolar vasoconstriction, possibly due to increased susceptibility to various stimuli. There is a major increase in peripheral resistance, reducing the capacity of the system and increasing diastolic pressure. Decreased renal blood flow causes an increase in renin, angiotensin, and aldosterone secretion. Resulting increases in vasoconstriction and blood volume further increase blood pressure. Chronic hypertension causes arterial wall damage, sclerosis, and stenosis. Aneurysms or atheromas may form, reducing blood flow to involved area. There is ischemia and necrosis of involved tissues. The areas most frequently damaged are the kidneys, brain, and retina. The end result of poorly controlled hypertension can be chronic renal failure, stroke, vision loss, or congestive heart failure.
91. It is often asymptomatic in the early stage, and initial symptoms are usually vague until complications arise.
92. Reduce salt intake, which reduces blood pressure; body weight, which, if reduced, puts less stress on the heart as it labors to pump blood through the circulatory system; fat tissue around the heart itself restricts the movement of the heart muscle; and stress, which lowers blood pressure and increase cardiovascular fitness, which strengthens the heart muscle.
93. patient compliance—*i.e.,* willingness to consistently follow treatment plan

ANTIHYPERTENSIVE MEDICATIONS

94. (Table 12.1)

Type of Antihypertensive	Mechanism of Action and Effects	Adverse Effects	Examples
Diuretics	Increased excretion of sodium and water, leading to decreased blood volume	Nausea, vomiting Orthostatic hypotension, dizziness Xerostomia Hypokalemia	Furosemide Hydrochlorothiazide
ACE inhibitors	Block formation of angiotensin II Decrease aldosterone secretion Prevent vasoconstriction	Headache Orthostatic hypotension, dizziness	Enalapril Ramipril Captopril Fosinopril
Calcium channel blockers	Vasodilation Decrease myocardial conduction and contractility	Dizziness, fainting, headache Orthostatic hypotension Constipation Gingival hypertension	Nifedipine Amlodipine Diltiazem
β-Adrenergic blockers	Prevent increased heart rate in response to sympathetic nervous system and cholamines	Bradycardia Dizziness, fatigue Orthostatic hypotension Sexual dysfunction	Metoprolol Atenolol Propranolol Nadolol

95. nausea, erectile dysfunction, orthostatic hypotension, dizziness
96.
    - platelet inhibitor: to prevent heart attacks and strokes
    - antihyperlidemic: to arrest or slow progression of atherosclerosis

PERIPHERAL VASCULAR DISEASE (PVD)

97.
    a. increasing fatigue and weakness in the legs
    b. intermittent claudication
    c. sensory impairment
    d. weak peripheral pulse distal to the occlusion
    e. marked pallor or cyanosis when legs elevated redness when they are dangling
    f. skin that is dry and hairless
    g. toenails that are thick and hard
    h. poorly perfused extremities that are cold
98.
    a. reduction in serum cholesterol levels
    b. platelet inhibitors or anticoagulants to reduce thrombosis
    c. smoking cessation

Copyright © 2027 by Elsevier, Inc. All rights are reserved, including those for text and data mining, AI training, and similar technologies.

d. exercise program
e. maintaining dependent position for the legs
f. peripheral vasodilators
g. surgical procedures to increase blood flow
h. preventive measures to avoid skin trauma
i. antibiotics for gangrenous ulcers
j. amputations when necessary to prevent infection spread; relieve pain

99. localized dilation of an arterial wall
100. Causes include atherosclerosis, trauma (particularly automobile accidents), syphilis, and congenital defects.
101. rupture, leading to moderate bleeding or severe hemorrhage and death; or thrombus may develop in the aneurysm, causing obstruction
102. inherent weakness or defect in vein walls or valves (familial tendency); long periods of standing
103.
    a. superficial varicosities on the legs appear as irregular, purplish, bulging veins in the legs
    b. edema in the feet
    c. fatigue and aching in the legs are common
    d. shiny, pigmented, and hairless skin
    e. ulcers may develop
104. *thrombophlebitis:* development of a thrombus in a vein in which inflammation is present; *phlebothrombosis:* spontaneous thrombus development in the absence of inflammation
105.
    a. blood stasis or sluggish blood flow
    b. endothelial injury
    c. increased blood coagulability
106.
    a. exercise
    b. elevation of legs
    c. compression or elastic stockings
107. (see also Chapter 13) Pulmonary embolus is a blood clot (or sometimes other material) that blocks a pulmonary artery or one of its branches. It typically originates in leg veins as a result of thrombophlebitis.

SHOCK

108. hypotension resulting from a decreased circulating blood volume, resulting in decreased tissue perfusion and general hypoxia
109.
    a. SNS and adrenal medulla stimulated to increase the heart rate, force of contractions, and systemic vasoconstriction
    b. renin secreted to activate angiotensin (a vasoconstrictor); aldosterone to increase blood volume (sodium and water retention)
    c. increased antidiuretic hormone (ADH) to promote water reabsorption in the kidneys and thereby increase blood volume
    d. glucocorticoids secreted to help stabilize the vascular system
    e. acidosis stimulates respirations, increasing oxygen supply
110. (Table 12.5)
    a. Thirst, anxiety, and restlessness occur, because the SNS is quickly stimulated by hypotension.
    b. Compensation follows, as vasoconstriction shunts blood from the viscera and skin to the vital areas.
    c. Progressive signs include lethargy, weakness, and faintness, and metabolic acidosis due to decrease in blood flow and blood pressure. Metabolic acidosis may result, as anaerobic metabolism increases lactic acid secretion.
111. If shock is prolonged, the body's responsiveness diminishes as oxygen supply decreases and wastes accumulate. Compensated metabolic acidosis progresses to decompensated acidosis (see also Chapter 6). There is depression of the central nervous system, loss of cell metabolism, and reduction in effectiveness of medications. The progression to irreversible shock results in acute renal failure due to tubular ischemia and necrosis and acute respiratory distress syndrome (ARDS).
112. (Emergency Treatment Box)
    a. Place patient in supine position
    b. Cover and keep warm
    c. Call 911 or other assistance
    d. Administer oxygen if possible
    e. Determine underlying cause and treat if possible (e.g., pressure for bleeding)
113.

Type of Shock	Etiology	Specific Manifestations	Specific Treatment
Hypovolemic or hemorrhagic	Blood or plasma loss Dehydration: vomiting, diarrhea "Third spacing"	Bleeding Burns Dysphagia, nausea, vomiting, diarrhea Ascites Signs of peritonitis	Blood or plasma transfusions Fluid and electrolyte replacement Treat specific cause (e.g., measures to stop bleeding)
Cardiogenic	Myocardial infarction Arrhythmias	Warning signs of infarction ECG changes	Antiarrhythmic agents ECG monitoring See treatment of myocardial infarction

Copyright © 2027 by Elsevier, Inc. All rights are reserved, including those for text and data mining, AI training, and similar technologies.

Type of Shock	Etiology	Specific Manifestations	Specific Treatment
Anaphylactic	Severe allergic or hypersensitivity reaction leads to generalized vasodilation	Severe dyspnea, wheezing, chest tightness Pruritus, urticaria (hives), tingling Flushing, feeling of warmth	Epinephrine IM or IV (Epi-Pen) Corticosteroids Antihistamines
Septic	Severe, overwhelming infection	High fever, possibly with chills Warm, flushed, dry skin Rapid, strong pulse Hyperventilation	Antibacterial Corticosteroids Antipyretics
Neurogenic (syncope)	Pain or fear Emotional upset (unpleasant sight or smell)	Sudden vertigo and loss of consciousness Flushed, warm skin	Spirits of ammonia "smelling salts" Lower head Remove stimulus

CONSOLIDATION

114.

i. right-sided heart failure
ii. thrombophlebitis
iii. myocardial infarction; arrhythmias
iv. rheumatic fever, endocarditis
v. thrombophlebitis
vi. heart failure
vii. congenital defects, rheumatic fever, rheumatic heart disease, tetralogy of Fallot, septal defects, valvular defects—stenosis and regurgitation
viii. myocardial infarction
ix. rheumatic fever
x. left-sided heart failure, mitral stenosis, mitral regurgitation

115. (Table 12.1)

i. antihypertensive, antiarrhythmic, prophylactic antianginal
ii. antianginal—prophylactic or acute
iii. scarlet fever, rheumatic fever, rheumatic heart disease
iv. antihypertensive antiarrhythmic, prophylactic antianginal
v. heart failure, antiarrhythmic
vi. heart failure, hypertension
vii. arrhythmias, post–myocardial infarction, rheumatic fever
viii. antihypertensive

116. Collateral circulation involves the development of alternative blood vessels that bypass narrowed or blocked coronary arteries, improving blood flow to the myocardium and reducing ischemia in coronary artery disease. Regular aerobic exercise, such as walking or cycling, promotes collateral vessel growth by increasing oxygen demand and stimulating angiogenesis.

117. The renin-angiotensin-aldosterone system (RAAS) is activated in congestive heart failure due to reduced cardiac output, leading to renin release, which forms angiotensin II, a potent vasoconstrictor that increases blood pressure and cardiac workload.

CHAPTER 13: Respiratory System Disorders

1. See Fig. 13.1 of the text.
   A. Upper respiratory system, B. Nasal cavity, C. Oral cavity, D. Tongue, E. Pharynx, F. Larynx (voice box), G. Lower respiratory system, H. Left lung, I. Left main bronchus, J. Pleura, K. Bronchiole, L. Diaphragm, M. Alveoli, N. Heart, O. Right lung, P. Right main bronchus, Q. Trachea, R. Epiglottis
2. See Fig. 13.7 of the text.
   A. Eupnea, B. Tachypnea, C. Bradypnea, D. Apnea, E. Hyperpnea, F. Cheyne-Stokes respiration, G. Ataxic breathing, H. Kussmaul's respiration, I. Apneusis, J. Obstructed breathing
3. (Fig. 13.8) otitis media, sinusitis, pneumonia
4. (Table 13.3)

	Croup (Laryngotracheobronchitis)	Epiglottitis	Bronchiolitis
Usual age	3 months to 3 years	3–7 years	2–12 months
Cause	Virus	*Haemophilus influenzae*	Virus: RSV
Onset	Gradual	Rapid	Gradual
Pathology	Inflammation of mucosa of larynx and trachea obstructs airway	Supraglottic inflammation and swelling of epiglottis obstruct airway	Inflammation of mucosa of bronchioles obstructs small passages

Copyright © 2027 by Elsevier, Inc. All rights are reserved,
including those for text and data mining, AI training, and similar technologies.

	Croup (Laryngotracheobronchitis)	Epiglottitis	Bronchiolitis
Significant signs and symptoms	Hoarse, barking cough Inspiratory stridor Restlessness	Drooling, dysphagia, high fever, appears ill, rapid respirations and pulse, tripod position at play	Increasing dyspnea, paroxysmal cough, wheezing, chest retractions, flared nostrils
Treatment	Cool, moisturized air from a humidifier, shower, or croup tent	Oxygen and antimicrobial therapy with intubation or tracheotomy if necessary	Supportive or symptomatic with monitoring of blood gases in severe cases

RSV, respiratory syncytial virus.

5. (Figs. 13.10 and 13.11, Table 13.4)

	Lobar Pneumonia	Bronchial Pneumonia	Interstitial Pneumonia
Causative agent	*Streptococcus pneumoniae*	Multiple bacteria	Influenza virus Mycoplasma
Onset	Sudden and acute	Insidious	Variable
Distribution within lungs	All of one or two lobes	Scattered small patches	Diffuse throughout lung
Pathophysiology	Inflammation of alveolar wall and leakage of cells, fibrin, and fluid into alveoli causing consolidation	Inflammation and purulent exudate in alveoli often arising from prior pooled secretions or irritation	Interstitial inflammation around alveoli Necrosis of bronchial epithelium
Signs and symptoms	High fever and chills Productive cough with rusty sputum Rales progressing to absence of breath sounds in affected lobes	Mild fever Productive cough with yellow-green sputum Dyspnea	Variable fever, headache Aching muscles Nonproductive hacking cough
Treatment	Antibacterial medication in combination with fluids; drugs to reduce fever; and oxygen Pneumococcal vaccine is recommended for the elderly and those at risk of other disease	Antibacterial medications	Erythromycin or tetracycline

6. *Pneumocystis carinii* pneumonia (PCP) is an atypical pneumonia that occurs as an opportunistic and often fatal infection in patients with AIDS. The etiological agent is a fungus that is inhaled and attaches to alveolar cells, causing necrosis and diffuse interstitial inflammation. Onset is marked by dyspnea and a nonproductive cough.
7. SARS-CoV (severe acute respiratory syndrome [SARS]-associated coronavirus) is the microbial agent responsible for SARS. It is transmitted by respiratory droplets during close contact.
8. Flulike symptoms are present for 3 to 7 days, followed several days later by a dry cough and marked dyspnea. By day 7, chest radiographs indicate spreading patchy areas of interstitial congestion and severe hypoxia; there may be thrombocytopenia, lymphopenia, and elevated liver enzymes (due to viral damage). The final stage is severe, sometimes fatal respiratory distress.
9. stage 1: fever, headache, myalgia, diarrhea; stage 2: nonproductive cough, severe dyspnea, hypoxia; stage 3: severe hypoxia, respiratory and metabolic acidosis
10. medications: ribavirin (antiviral) and GC-methylprednisolone; oxygen with mechanical ventilation
11. Unique pathophysiological characteristics include rapid and firm attachment of the virus to lung cells and the triggering of a cytokine storm (see Chapter 7) particularly in older patients (60 and older) as well as immunocompromised individuals and patients with serious underlying conditions.
12. The **molecular tests** are looking for COVID-19 genetic material. PCR (polymerase chain reaction) method is used to amplify nucleic acids present in a sample. Reverse transcription polymerase is then used to determine whether the nucleic acid amplified by PCR matches the COVID-19 genetics. **Antigen tests** are looking for the presence of viral antigens.

Copyright © 2027 by Elsevier, Inc. All rights are reserved, including those for text and data mining, AI training, and similar technologies.

These are often called rapid COVID-19 tests as they can be done at home and produce quick results. These tests are relatively accurate but not as accurate as the PCR molecular tests which are done by health care professionals in a laboratory environment. The antigen test may not detect the disease if it is in the early stages and the person is showing no symptoms. If an antigen test is negative, it is recommended the person takes another antigen test after 48 hours.

13. A number of drugs have been used for therapeutic and/or prophylactic use, including the malaria drug hydroxyquinoline combined with antibiotics and remdesivir, a broad-spectrum antiviral drug. At this writing, the FDA approved drugs for treating COVID-19 patients include: Paxlovid, remdesivir (Veklury), baricitinib (Olumiant), and tocilizumab (Actemra).
14. It is difficult to control the spread of an unidentified causative agent because the type of microbe has not been identified as bacterial, viral, or fungal. The routes of transmission may not be known. The agent's sensitivity to antimicrobial medications is not known. The usual course of the infection (*i.e.,* complications and prognosis) may not be known.

TUBERCULOSIS

15. acid-fast, aerobic, slow-growing bacillus that is resistant to drying and many disinfectants
16. The cell wall prevents digestion and destruction by defensive cells.
17. Individuals who are at high risk of contracting tuberculosis (TB) are those whose resistance is lowered because of immunodeficiency, malnutrition, alcoholism, conditions of war, or chronic disease. There may be a genetic susceptibility. Children are vulnerable, as are the homeless. Patients with AIDS are also at high risk.
18. (Figs. 13.12 and 13.13) In the primary infection, the pathogen is engulfed by macrophages and causes local inflammatory reaction, usually on the periphery of the upper lobe. Some bacilli migrate to the lymph nodes, activating a type IV hypersensitivity response. Lymphocytes and macrophages cluster to form a granuloma at the site of inflammation. The granuloma contains the bacilli, some of which remain alive, forming a tubercle. Caseation necrosis develops in the center of the tubercle. The secondary infection is the active infection. It often arises years after primary infection as a result of decreased host resistance. Tissue necrosis and cavitation occur, forming a large open area in the lung and erosion into the bronchi and blood vessels. Hemoptysis is common. Infection may spread to other body systems, and bacilli may infect sputum.
19. Ghon tubercle is the core of caseation necrosis, surrounded by lymphocytes and macrophages. It is eventually walled off by fibrous tissue and usually becomes calcified.
20. Primary TB is asymptomatic. Secondary infection has an insidious onset with vague symptoms of anorexia, malaise, fatigue, and weight loss; afternoon low-grade fever and night sweats; prolonged and increasingly severe cough; and productive, purulent sputum, often containing blood.
21. rapidly progressive form in which multiple granulomas affect large areas of the lungs with rapid dissemination via the bloodstream; resistant to treatment
22. with chest x-ray, acid staining of sputum specimen, and sputum culture
23. (See Chapter 3, Type IV Delayed Hypersensitivity) The Mantoux test is the tuberculin test. A positive skin test does NOT mean the person has active TB. It means that there has been adequate exposure to cause a hypersensitivity reaction.
24. isoniazid (INH); rifampin; ethambutol; pyrazinamide; streptomycin; multiple drugs required to prevent the development of resistant strains; 3 months to 1 year or possibly longer, depending on the health of the individual (e.g., someone who also has full-blown AIDS will probably take TB medications for the rest of his or her life).
25. An individual will become noncontagious when sputum is negative for microbes, usually about 1 to 2 months. Drugs are prescribed for a longer period of time to ensure eradication of the infection.
26.
    - those whose skin test has converted from negative to positive within the past 2 years
    - those who have radiographic changes consistent with TB, even if their sputum is negative
    - anyone who is living with, or has frequent close contact with, an individual with active TB
    - individuals who have immunosuppression due to disease or medications
    - people who are HIV positive or have full-blown AIDS
    - people with hematological cancer
27. Isoniazid, rifampin, ethambutol, pyrazinamide, and streptomycin; usually prescribed for 6 months to 1 year
28. (Think About) Have regular skin tests and, if the test is positive, regular chest radiographs; maintain host resistance (get adequate rest and nutrition).
29. (Think About)
    - What was the date of the skin test?
    - Was he vaccinated against TB as a child?
    - Has he had any known contact with a person who has TB or a history of TB?
    - Did he have a follow-up chest radiograph or sputum specimen for an acid-fast bacilli (AFB) test?
    - Did the doctor prescribe medication?
    - Is he taking the medication? How long has he been taking the medication?
30.
    - Was TB actually diagnosed, or was it a positive skin test?
    - Was he prescribed medications?
    - How long were the medications prescribed for?
    - Did he actually take the medication at the intervals and for the time period prescribed?
    - When was his last chest radiograph?

Copyright © 2027 by Elsevier, Inc. All rights are reserved,
including those for text and data mining, AI training, and similar technologies.

CYSTIC FIBROSIS

31. (See Chapter 7, Table 7.1) an autosomal recessive inherited disorder
32. (See Chapter 7, Fig. 7.4) Both parents are heterozygous (*i.e.,* carriers of cystic fibrosis CF). There is a 25% probability that the baby's siblings will have *CF.*
33. (See Chapter 7, Fig. 7.4) There is a 50% probability that the child will have CF and a 50% probability that he will be a carrier.
34. (Fig. 13.14) Cystic fibrosis is a common genetic disorder involving a protein in chloride ion transport in cell membranes. This defect in the exocrine glands causes thick secretions, such as tenacious mucus. Primary effects are seen in lungs and pancreas where mucus blocks passages. In the lungs, there is progressive destruction of lung tissue and atelectasis, and infections are common. Bronchiectasis and emphysematous changes develop. Eventually, respiratory failure or cor pulmonale develops. In the digestive tract, the first indication of abnormality may be meconium ileus in newborns. Pancreatic blockage leads to digestive enzyme deficit in the intestines. Malabsorption and malnutrition develop. Potential pancreatic glandular tissue damage results in diabetes mellitus in some individuals. Biliary obstruction leads to fat and fat-soluble vitamin malabsorption and deficiencies. Ultimately, the general state of malabsorption, malnutrition, and dehydration develops. The salivary glands are mildly affected, causing patchy fibrosis. Sweat glands are affected, producing high chloride sweat and potential electrolyte disturbance in hot weather or during strenuous exercise. Obstructions in male (vas deferens) and female (cervix) reproductive systems lead to sterility or infertility.
35. meconium ileus at birth; salty skin; signs of malabsorption: steatorrhea, abdominal distention, and failure to gain weight; chronic cough and frequent respiratory infections; progressive hypoxia, fatigue, and exercise intolerance; growth failure
36. electrolyte analysis of sweat; stool analysis for fat content and trypsin; pulmonary function tests, radiographs, and blood gases; genetic analysis
37. interdisciplinary team approach; replacement therapy for pancreatic enzymes and bile salts; specialized diet; measures to avoid dehydration; chest physiotherapy; bronchodilators and humidifiers; aggressive treatment of infections; oxygen therapy for advanced disease
38. With treatment, individuals with CF, on average, live into early adulthood. Death is usually brought on through respiratory infections and respiratory or heart failure.

LUNG CANCER

39. Venous return and lymphatics bring tumor cells from many distant sites to the heart and then into the pulmonary circulation.
40. cigarette smoking, especially heavy smokers; secondhand smoke; chronic obstructive pulmonary disease (COPD); genetic factors; occupational or industrial exposure to carcinogens
41. obstruction of airflow by tumor growth into the bronchus; inflammation surrounding the tumor stimulates cough and predisposes secondary infection; pleural effusion, hemothorax, pneumothorax due to inflammation or erosion of pleura; paraneoplastic syndrome; general systemic effects of cancer
42. Early signs related to respiratory involvement include persistent productive cough, dyspnea, and wheezing; radiographic changes signifying pneumonia; hemoptysis; pleural involvement—effusion; pneumothorax or hemothorax; chest pain; hoarseness; facial or arm edema and headache due to compression of superior vena cava; dysphagia; and atelectasis. Systemic signs include weight loss, anemia, and fatigue. Paraneoplastic syndrome is indicated by signs of specific endocrine disorder. Signs of metastasis depend on site (e.g., bone).
43.
    - surgical resection or lobectomy
    - chemotherapy
    - radiation
    - photodynamic therapy

ASPIRATION

44. passage of food or fluid, vomitus, drugs, or other foreign material into the trachea and lungs
45. young children; children with congenital anomalies such as cleft palate; any individual with depressed swallowing or gag reflex (e.g., following anesthesia or stroke or comatose patients); individuals who eat or drink while lying down or talk while eating
46.

    Solid objects lodge in the airway and totally block airflow at that place.

    Large objects may occlude the trachea and block all airflow.

    Solid objects lodging in a bronchus lead to nonaeration and collapse of the area distal to the obstruction (see Fig. 13.24C).

    Ball-valve effect of solid object: air flows in on inspiration, airway closes on expiration.

    Swelling of some foods (beans) causes them to become more firmly lodged.

    Sharp, pointed objects, like bone fragments, may traumatize mucosa and cause inflammation that further adds to the airway barrier.

    Fatty or irritating solids, such as peanuts, cause inflammation, creating edema and further impeding airflow.

    Irritating liquids (e.g., vomitus, alcohol) cause severe inflammation, narrowing airways, and can increase secretions; if alveoli are involved, gaseous exchange may be impaired: this is called chemical or *aspiration* pneumonia.

    Complications include respiratory distress syndrome, pulmonary abscess, and systemic effects of aspirated solvents.
47. coughing and choking with marked dyspnea; stridor and hoarseness (upper airway obstruction); wheezing (liquids); tachycardia and tachypnea; nasal flaring,

Copyright © 2027 by Elsevier, Inc. All rights are reserved, including those for text and data mining, AI training, and similar technologies.

chest retractions; inability to speak or make a sound (total obstruction of larynx or trachea)

48. (See Emergency Treatment for Aspiration) Stand behind the victim with encircling arms, position a fist, thumb side against the abdomen, just below the sternum, place the other hand over the fist, and thrust forcefully inward and upward.

ASTHMA

49. a disease that involves periodic episodes of severe but reversible bronchial obstruction
50. Extrinsic asthma involves acute episodes triggered by a type I hypersensitivity reaction to an inhaled antigen. A familial history of other allergies is common. Onset usually occurs in children. Intrinsic asthma usually occurs in adulthood. Other types of stimuli target hyperresponsive tissues in the airway, initiating the acute attack. These stimuli include respiratory infections, exposure to cold, exercise, certain drugs such as aspirin, stress, and inhalation of irritants such as cigarette smoke.
51. (Fig. 13.18) an acute allergic response to stimuli affecting the bronchioles, resulting in inflammation of the mucosa with edema, contraction of smooth muscle (bronchoconstriction), and increased thick mucus secretion in the air passages, with resulting airway obstruction and interference with airflow and oxygen supply
52.
   - hyperinflation of the lung, with increased residual volume
   - atelectasis
   - respiratory and metabolic acidosis
   - status asthmaticus
   - chronic asthma and obstructive lung disease
53.
   - cough, dyspnea, tightness in the chest, and agitation as airway obstruction increases; cannot talk
   - wheezing
   - rapid and labored breathing
   - coughing up thick and tenacious mucus
   - tachycardia and perhaps pulsus paradoxus
   - hypoxia
   - respiratory alkalosis, initially due to hyperventilation
   - respiratory acidosis, in time, due to air trapping
   - marked fatigue causes reduced respiratory effort and weaker cough
   - metabolic acidosis
   - severe respiratory distress; hypoventilation leading to hypoxemia and respiratory acidosis
   - respiratory failure: decreasing responsiveness, cyanosis
54.
   - avoidance of triggering stimuli
   - a program of desensitization or "allergy shots" for allergens that cannot be avoided (e.g., house dust)
   - good ventilation: at home, school, work
   - conditioning exercises to strengthen muscles of respiration and improve cardiovascular fitness (swimming is particularly good as long as the water is not too cold)
   - relaxation techniques to help cope with stressful situations and hopefully to avoid precipitating an attack
   - prophylactic medications, such as flu vaccinations or inoculations
   - avoidance of individuals with respiratory infections
55.

Drug Group	Action and Effects	Adverse Effects	Example and Route
Bronchodilators	Relax bronchial smooth muscle, leading to bronchodilation	Tachycardia, palpitations, CNS stimulation: tremors, insomnia Stinging sensation in mouth	Inhalants: albuterol or salbutamol (Ventolin) metaproterenol (Alupent)
Corticosteroids	Decrease inflammation Decrease the immune response (hypersensitivity)	Oral fungal (candidal) infections with inhalants Cushing's with oral administration	Inhalation: beclomethasone (Beclovent) Oral: prednisone
Histamine release inhibitors	Inhibit release of histamine from sensitized mast cells Decrease the number of eosinophils	Rare	Inhalation: cromolyn (Intal)
Leukotriene receptor antagonists	Block inflammatory response to prevent bronchoconstriction and mucus production	GI distress occurs rarely	Inhalation: montelukast (Singulair) zafirlukast (Accolade)

56. Bronchodilators can be used during an acute asthmatic attack because their mechanism of action is to relax bronchial smooth muscle with minimal effects on the heart.
57.
   - How frequent are his asthmatic attacks?
   - When was the last one?
   - What are the triggering stimuli for an acute episode?

Copyright © 2027 by Elsevier, Inc. All rights are reserved, including those for text and data mining, AI training, and similar technologies.

- How long do they usually last?
- What is the treatment he uses during bronchospasm?
- Has he had any emergencies when he had to seek medical help?

CHRONIC OBSTRUCTIVE PULMONARY DISEASE (COPD)

58. (Table 13.5) Smoking is the leading causative factor. Contributing factors include cystic fibrosis and bronchiectasis; many occupational lung diseases such as silicosis, asbestosis, farmer's lung, and industrial/urban pollution.
59. Both conditions are characterized by hypoxia—this stimulates release of erythropoietin by the kidneys, which in turn stimulates increased production of red blood cells.
60. destruction of pulmonary alveolar walls and septa, leading to large permanently inflated alveolar air spaces
61.
    - loss of surface area for gas exchange
    - loss of pulmonary capillaries, affecting perfusion and diffusion of gases
    - loss of elasticity, affecting ability of lung to recoil on expiration
    - altered ventilation-perfusion ratio
    - decreased support for other pulmonary structures such as the small bronchi, leading to further collapse and obstruction of airflow during expiration
62. Hyperventilation is a compensatory mechanism that alone helps maintain adequate oxygen levels until late in the disease; therefore, the patient's color is normal (*i.e.,* pink), unlike in many respiratory disorders that are characterized by hypoxia and cyanosis.
63.
    - barrel chest
    - pneumothorax
    - frequent infections
    - pulmonary hypertension and cor pulmonale
    - clubbed fingers
    - secondary polycythemia
64. Hypercapnia develops, resulting in respiratory acidosis. Hypoxia leads to metabolic acidosis. Blood pH decreases.
65. Hypoxia becomes the driving force for respiration as respiratory control adapts to chronic hypercapnia.
66. Barrel chest refers to the hyperinflation of lungs that leads to increased anterior-posterior diameter of chest. The chest appears like a barrel. The condition develops because accessory muscles of expiration hypertrophy.
67.
    - avoidance of respiratory irritants and sources of infections
    - smoking cessation
    - immunization against influenza and pneumonia
    - pulmonary rehabilitation
    - nutrition counseling: maintenance of adequate nutrition and hydration
    - bronchodilators, antimicrobials, and oxygen therapy when needed
    - lung reduction surgery
68. Following chronic irritation of the bronchi, the mucosa is inflamed and swollen; there is hypertrophy and hyperplasia of the mucous glands and increased secretions and fibrosis and thickening of the bronchial wall and further obstruction. Secretions pool distal to the obstruction and are difficult to remove; oxygen levels are low; and cyanosis may occur during coughing episodes.
69. constant productive cough
70. Hypoxia is characteristic feature, particularly during coughing episodes. This results in poor color or cyanosis. Pulmonary congestion and cor pulmonale also commonly occur with chronic bronchitis, resulting in peripheral edema. Thus there is a designation as a "blue bloater" as opposed to someone with emphysema, a "pink puffer."
71. Treatments include reducing exposure to irritants, prompt treatment of infections, influenza and pneumonia vaccination, and use of expectorants, bronchodilators, chest therapy, low-flow oxygen, and nutritional supplementation.
72. (Table 13.5)

	Asthma	**Emphysema**	**Chronic Bronchitis**
Etiology and predisposing factor	Family history of allergies Air pollution Sedentary lifestyle Obesity	Smoking Air pollution Genetic factors	Smoking Air pollution
Location	Small bronchi, bronchioles	Alveoli	Bronchi
Pathophysiology	Inflammation, bronchoconstriction, increased mucus production, obstruction, repeat attacks lead to damage	Destruction of alveolar walls, loss of elasticity, impaired expiration, barrel chest, hyperinflation	Increased mucous glands and secretions, inflammation and infection, obstruction
Signs and symptoms	Cough, dyspnea, wheezing, thick, tenacious mucus	Some coughing, marked dyspnea	Early constant unproductive cough, some dyspnea

Copyright © 2027 by Elsevier, Inc. All rights are reserved, including those for text and data mining, AI training, and similar technologies.

	Asthma	Emphysema	Chronic Bronchitis
Complications	Cyanosis if status asthmaticus	Some infections Cor pulmonale: sometimes, late	Cyanosis; frequent infections Cor pulmonale
Treatments	Avoidance of triggering stimuli A program of desensitization or "allergy shots" for allergens that cannot be avoided (e.g., house dust) Good ventilation: at home, school, work Conditioning exercises to strengthen muscles of respiration and improve cardiovascular fitness Fitness (swimming is particularly good as long as the water is not too cold) Relaxation techniques to help cope with stressful situations and hopefully to avoid precipitating an attack Flu vaccinations or inoculations Avoidance of individuals with respiratory infections	Avoidance of respiratory irritants and sources of infections Smoking cessation Immunization against influenza and pneumonia Pulmonary rehabilitation Nutrition counseling: maintenance of adequate nutrition and hydration Bronchodilators, antimicrobials, and oxygen therapy when needed Lung reduction surgery	Reducing exposure to irritants Prompt treatment of infections Influenza and pneumonia vaccination Use of expectorants, bronchodilators Chest physiotherapy Low-flow oxygen and nutritional supplementation

73. Bronchiectasis is an irreversible abnormal dilation of the bronchi. Dilations can be saccular or elongated. This condition can be caused by cystic fibrosis or COPD.
74. Pneumonoconiosis is a chronic restrictive disease resulting from long-term exposure to irritating particles such as asbestos. Treatment involves identifying and ending exposure to the damaging agent.

PULMONARY EDEMA

75. Causes include inflammation in the lungs, increasing capillary permeability; plasma protein levels are low, decreasing plasma osmotic pressure; pulmonary hypertension, increasing hydrostatic pressure.
76. (Fig. 13.22) Pulmonary edema occurs when excess fluid develops in the alveolar tissue. This fluid interferes with gaseous exchange, leading to severe hypoxemia. This accumulation of fluid interferes with the action of surfactant, leading to difficulty in expansion of lungs, which ultimately collapse.
77. Signs and symptoms include cough, orthopnea, and rales; hemoptysis as congestion increases; frothy sputum; dyspnea; cyanosis due to increasing hypoxemia.
78. Sputum becomes frothy when air mixes with secretions and becomes blood-tinged as a result of ruptured capillaries in the lungs.
79. When the individual is placed in a supine position, the fluid that has accumulated in the bases of the lungs starts to shift into the upper lobes. Venous return to the heart and lungs is increased when in a supine position. The individual feels a sense of suffocation. This is called orthopnea.
80. Causative factors must be treated and supportive care such as oxygen therapy is provided; positive pressure mechanical ventilation may be necessary in severe cases. Upper body is elevated. Diuretics may be given to reduce fluid.

PULMONARY EMBOLUS

81. a blood clot or mass of material that obstructs the pulmonary artery or a branch of it
82. Most pulmonary emboli originate in the deep veins, primarily in the legs. Other potential sources include fat emboli from the bone marrow (fractures), vegetations resulting from endocarditis, amniotic fluid emboli, and tumor cell emboli.
83.
    - bedridden patients who have been immobile for long periods (e.g., hospitalized patients)
    - anyone with leg trauma
    - mothers during childbirth
    - patients with congestive heart failure
    - patients with dehydration or increased coagulability of the blood
    - patients who have cancer
    - airplane or automobile passengers who remain seated for prolonged periods of time
84. (Fig. 13.23) The effects depend on the size and location of the embolism. Small pulmonary emboli are frequently "silent" or asymptomatic. Multiple small emboli, however, equal the effect of a large embolus. Moderate-sized emboli usually cause respiratory impairment. Large emboli affect the cardiovascular system, causing right-sided heart failure and shock. Sudden death often occurs.
85. With a small embolus, symptoms include transient chest pain, cough, or dyspnea. With a larger embolus, symptoms include chest pain that increases with coughing or deep breathing, and tachypnea and dyspnea develop suddenly; later, hemoptysis and fever, anxiety and restlessness, pallor, and tachycardia

Copyright © 2027 by Elsevier, Inc. All rights are reserved, including those for text and data mining, AI training, and similar technologies.

occur. A massive emboli is characterized by severe crushing chest pain, low blood pressure, rapid, weak pulse, and loss of consciousness. Fat emboli are distinguished by development of acute respiratory distress, petechial rash on the trunk, and neurological signs such as confusion and disorientation.

86. heparin or fibrinolytic agent

EXPANSION DISORDERS

87. (Fig. 13.24)

	Atelectasis	**Bronchiectasis**
Definition	Nonaeration or collapse of a lung or part of a lung	Irreversible dilation or widening of bronchi with damage to smooth muscle and pooling of secretions
Etiology	Total obstruction of an airway Compression of airway Increased alveolar surface tension Fibrotic tissue in lungs or pleura Following anesthesia or prolonged bed rest	Complication of: Cystic fibrosis COPD Childhood infections Aspiration of foreign bodies
Complications	Permanent lung damage	Recurrent lung infections
Signs and symptoms	Dyspnea; increased respirations Tachycardia Chest pain Abnormal chest expansion Tracheal shift	Chronic productive cough Purulent sputum Rales and rhonchi Dyspnea, hemoptysis Foul breath Weight loss, anemia, fatigue

88. (Table 13.7, Fig. 13.25)

	Pleural Effusion	**Pneumothorax**
Definition	Excessive fluid in pleural cavity	Air in pleural cavity
Etiology	Inflammation or secondary to tumor in lung or chest wall	Spontaneous Rupture of a bleb (emphysema) Erosion by tumor Cavitation due to TB Puncture wound (broken rib, gunshot, knife wound)
Signs and symptoms	Dyspnea Chest pain Increased heart and respiratory rates Absence of breath sounds in affected area	Increased, labored respirations with dyspnea Pain Asymmetrical chest movements Tachycardia

89. (Fig. 13.26) Flail chest results from fractures of the thorax (usually from falls and automobile accidents)—usually includes fractures of three to six ribs in two places or fracture of the sternum and a number of consecutive ribs resulting in *paradoxical movement* during inspiration and *mediastinal flutter* if injury is extensive.

90. Causes of acute respiratory failure include chronic conditions such as emphysema, combination of a chronic with an acute disorder such as emphysema complicated by pneumonia or pneumothorax, acute respiratory disorders such as chest trauma, pulmonary embolus, or acute asthma, and many neuromuscular diseases such as myasthenia gravis, amyotrophic lateral sclerosis (ALS), and muscular dystrophy.

91.

	Infant Respiratory Distress Syndrome	**Adult Respiratory Distress Syndrome**
Etiology	Premature birth resulting in decreased surfactant	Systemic sepsis Prolonged shock Burns and smoke inhalation Aspiration Near-drowning

Copyright © 2027 by Elsevier, Inc. All rights are reserved, including those for text and data mining, AI training, and similar technologies.

	Infant Respiratory Distress Syndrome	Adult Respiratory Distress Syndrome
Pathophysiology	Lungs collapse with each expiration, resulting in diffuse atelectasis, poor lung perfusion, and increased alveolar capillary permeability, causing fluid and fibrin to leak into alveoli that decreases lung expansion and gas exchange	Damage to surfactant-producing cells and increased capillary permeability, leading to diffuse atelectasis and decreased tidal volume and vital capacity and fluid accumulation in lungs, all of which predispose to pneumonia
Signs and symptoms	Respirations greater than 60/minute Nasal flaring; chest retractions Decreased blood pressure, cyanosis, depressed responsiveness Apnea	Marked dyspnea Tachycardia Decreased partial pressure of oxygen (Po_2) Rales Frothy sputum Cyanosis Lethargy
Treatment	Corticosteroids to mother during labor Synthetic surfactant Mechanical ventilation and O_2	Treat underlying cause Mechanical ventilation and O_2

92.

a) air in the pleural cavity; iii. pneumothorax
b) abnormal widening of the bronchi; iv. bronchiectasis
c) excessive fluid in pleural cavity; i. pleural effusion
d) chronic disorder resulting from continued exposure to irritating particles; vi. pneumoconiosis
e) fungal infection of the lungs; v. histoplasmosis
f) collapse of a portion of the lung; ii. atelectasis

CONSOLIDATION

93.

a. asthma
b. pulmonary edema
c. pulmonary edema
d. emphysema
e. TB
f. asthma
g. *Pneumocystis carinii* pneumonia
h. cystic fibrosis
i. atelectasis
j. chronic bronchitis
k. pulmonary embolus
l. adult respiratory distress syndrome
m. pneumothorax
n. cystic fibrosis
o. cystic fibrosis
p. tuberculosis
q. bronchiectasis
r. pleurisy
s. TB
t. asthma

CHAPTER 14: Nervous System Disorders

ACUTE DISORDERS

1. See Fig. 14.3 of the text. *Anatomical Features:*
   A. Motor cortex, B. Central sulcus, C. Sensory cortex, D. Parietal lobe, E. Occipital lobe, F. Visual association, G. Cerebellum, H. Medulla, I. Pons, J. Temporal lobe, K. Lateral sulcus, L. Frontal lobe, M. Premotor cortex. *Functional Features:* N. Intellect Personality, O. Broca's Speech Area, V. Wernicke's Area, P. Auditory Area, Q. Memory, T. Balance Equilibrium Coordination, R. RAS, S. Vital Centers, U. Visual Area.
2. dura mater: outer layer; subdural space: beneath the dura; arachnoid; subarachnoid space: below the arachnoid—contains cerebrospinal fluid (CSF); pia mater: closest to the brain
3. The CSF provides a cushion for the brain and spinal cord and is produced by the choroid plexuses located in the ventricles.
4. i. Acetylcholine (ACh), ii. ACh, iii. PNS is ACh, SNS is norepinephrine
5. (Table 14.4)
   i. increased heart rate
   ii. secretion of epinephrine and norepinephrine
   iii. bronchodilation
   iv. pupil dilation
   v. decreased
6. cerebral cortex and the reticular activating system (RAS) in the brainstem
7. cessation of brain function (e.g., flat or inactive EEG), absence of brainstem reflexes or responses, absence of spontaneous respirations without ventilator assistance, certainty of irreversible brain damage by confirmation of the cause of the dysfunction

Copyright © 2027 by Elsevier, Inc. All rights are reserved, including those for text and data mining, AI training, and similar technologies.

8. (Table 14.6) Aphasia refers to an inability to comprehend or express language. Types:
   i. Expressive, or motor aphasia: impaired ability to speak or write fluently or appropriately
      Areas of the brain affected: Broca's area of frontal lobe, inferior motor cortex
   ii. Receptive, or sensory aphasia: inability to read or understand the spoken word
      Area of brain affected: Wernicke's area in the left temporal lobe
   iii. Global aphasia: generally describes a combination of expressive and receptive aphasia
      Areas of the brain affected: any major damage to the brain including Broca's and Wernicke's areas and communicating fibers
9. (Fig. 14.8; Table 14.7) brain hemorrhage, trauma, cerebral edema, infection, tumors, or accumulation of excessive amounts of CSF
10. (Table 14.7)
    - increase in pressure in the brain
    - decrease in arterial blood flood into the "high pressure" area
    - pressure increases at the site of the problem initially but gradually is dispersed throughout the CNS
    - brain compression
    - decrease in functionality of neurons, both locally and generally
    - brain death
11. (Fig. 14.8; Table 14.7)
    Early manifestations:
    - decreasing level of consciousness or responsiveness (lethargy); pressure on RAS (brainstem) or cerebral cortex
    - severe headache; stretching or distortion of meninges or walls of large blood vessels
    - vomiting; pressure on emetic center in medulla
    - increasing blood pressure with increasing pulse pressure; Cushing's reflex, response to cerebral ischemia causes systemic vasoconstriction
    - slow heart rate; response to increasing blood pressure
    - papilledema; increased pressure of CSF causes swelling around the optic disc
    - pupil becomes fixed and dilated on ipsilateral side of lesion initially; eventually, both pupils become fixed and dilated; pressure on cranial nerve III (oculomotor)

Tumors

12. signs of increased intracranial pressure, often beginning with morning headaches that increase in severity and frequency; vomiting; and lethargy and irritability; focal or generalized seizures may be the first sign

TIAs and CVAs

13. temporary localized reduction of blood flow in the brain
14. The manifestations of a transient ischemic attack (TIA) are directly related to the location of the ischemia. The patient remains conscious. Intermittent short episodes of impaired function, such as muscle weakness in an arm or leg, visual disturbances, or numbness and paresthesia in the face, may occur. Transient aphasia or confusion may develop. The attack may last a few minutes or longer but rarely lasts more than 1 to 2 hours, and then the signs disappear.
15. They warn of the potential development of an obstruction related to atherosclerosis that may lead to a cerebrovascular event (stroke).
16. TIAs do not cause permanent brain damage; a stroke (cerebrovascular accident [CVA]) does. TIAs are caused by partial arterial obstruction or spasm; strokes (CVAs) are caused by total obstruction or hemorrhage.
17. Individuals with:
    - diabetes
    - hypertension (especially if chronic, severe in the elderly)
    - systemic lupus erythematosus
    - elevated cholesterol levels (hypercholesterolemia)
    - hyperlipidemia
    - atherosclerosis
    - history of TIAs
    - increasing age
    - obstructive sleep apnea
    - heart disease
    - combination of oral contraceptives and cigarette smoking
18. (Warning Signs Box 14.1); The warning signs of a stroke and TIA are often identical because both involve ischemia to specific brain regions, producing focal deficits based on the affected area. The key difference lies in the duration and reversibility of symptoms, with TIAs being transient and strokes causing lasting damage.
    - sudden transient weakness, numbness, or tingling in the face, an arm or leg, or on one side of the body
    - temporary loss of speech, failure to comprehend, or confusion
    - sudden loss of vision
    - sudden severe headache
    - unusual dizziness or unsteadiness
19.
    i. occlusion of an artery by an atheroma (most common)
    ii. embolism lodging in the cerebral artery
    iii. intracerebral hemorrhage
20. (Fig. 14.13) Infarction of brain tissue results from lack of blood; tissue necrosis results from total occlusion of a cerebral blood vessel or the consequence of a ruptured cerebral vessel. Within 5 minutes of ischemia, irreversible cell damage occurs. A central area of necrosis develops, surrounded by an area of inflammation. As time passes, the tissue liquefies, leaving a cavity. The cerebral edema increases the neurological deficits. As the edema decreases, functions performed by the inflamed area start to return.

Copyright © 2027 by Elsevier, Inc. All rights are reserved, including those for text and data mining, AI training, and similar technologies.

21. (Table 14.8)

	Thrombus CVA	Embolus CVA	Hemorrhage CVA
Predisposing factors	Atherosclerosis	Atherosclerosis Left ventricular MI Rheumatic heart disease Valvular disease Prosthetic heart valves Endocarditis Arrhythmias Heart failure	Hypertension
Onset	Gradual May be preceded by TIAs Often at rest	Sudden	Sudden
Effects	Localized	Localized	Widespread Increased ICP Often fatal
Immediate treatment	Fibrinolytic agents—"clot buster"	Fibrinolytic agents Thrombectomy	Ligation of ruptured vessel if accessible
Prognosis	Depends on size and location of injury, plus speed of initiation of treatment	Depends on size and location of injury, plus speed of initiation of treatment	Depends on size and location of injury, plus speed of initiation of treatment Worst prognosis—most often fatal

CVA, cerebrovascular accident; *ICP*, intracranial pressure; *MI*, myocardial infarction; *TIA*, transient ischemic attack.

22.
- MI in left side of heart: rheumatic heart disease, endocarditis, valvular disease, prosthetic heart valves, left-sided heart failure, arrhythmias
- carotid arteries

23.
- because damage much more widespread—often increased intracranial pressure (ICP)
- both hemispheres involved
- sudden onset—no time for development of collateral circulation
- secondary effects of bleeding: vasospasm, electrolyte imbalances, acidosis, cellular edema

24. Manifestations depend on location of the obstruction, size of artery involved, and the functional area affected. However, the four general types of deficits include:
    i. motor deficits: contralateral muscle weakness or paralysis (hemiplegia)
    ii. sensory deficits: contralateral paresthesia or numbness; possibly loss of vision
    iii. speech deficits: aphasia when the dominant side of the brain is involved
    iv. cognitive and emotional manifestations: confusion, loss of problem-solving skills, personality changes, impairment of spatial relationships

25.
- medications: depend on underlying problem
- antihypertensives
- platelet inhibitors or anticoagulants
- glucocorticoids
- physiotherapy
- occupational therapy
- speech therapy

26. loss of movement and sensation on the right side of the body (contralateral); expressive or motor aphasia

Aneurysms

27. (Fig. 14.14) localized dilation in an artery; cerebral aneurysms are often multiple and usually occur at the points of bifurcation on the circle of Willis
28. increased blood pressure, for example, during exertion
29. Enlarging aneurysm may cause pressure on the surrounding structures, such as the optic chiasm or cranial nerves, resulting in visual disturbances and headaches as tension increases on the vessel wall and meninges. Small leaks cause headaches, photophobia, and periods of confusion, slurred speech, or weakness. Nuchal rigidity may develop. Massive ruptures result in immediate severe headaches, vomiting, photophobia, and perhaps seizures or loss of consciousness. Death may occur shortly after rupture.

Copyright © 2027 by Elsevier, Inc. All rights are reserved, including those for text and data mining, AI training, and similar technologies.

Infections

30.

	Meningitis	Encephalitis
Causative agents	Meningococci *Escherichia coli* Influenza Pneumococci	Western equine virus West Nile virus Herpes simplex
Predisposing factors	Other infections (sinusitis, otitis, mumps, measles) Abscessed tooth Head trauma or surgery	Insect bites
Pathophysiology	Increased ICP Edema of arachnoid and pia maters Purulent exudates that cover brain surface and is in CSF	Infection involves tissue of brain and cord, especially basal ganglia May include meninges Necrosis and inflammation may lead to permanent damage
Manifestations	Sudden onset Severe headache, back pain, photophobia Nuchal rigidity Vomiting Irritability, lethargy, stupor, or seizures Fever and chills Leukocytosis	Severe headache Stiff neck Vomiting Lethargy Seizures Fever Change in neurological function Decreasing level of consciousness
Treatment	Appropriate antimicrobial agent	Antiviral agent if available Supportive measures

CSF, cerebrospinal fluid; *ICP,* intracranial pressure.

31. Varicella-zoster virus—occurs years after the primary infection, the chickenpox (usually occurs in childhood). It typically manifests in adults, especially older individuals or those with weakened immune systems (e.g., due to stress, aging, or illness), when the dormant virus in nerve ganglia reactivates, causing a painful rash along a nerve pathway.
32. The cause of Reye syndrome has not yet been fully determined, but it is linked to a viral infection, such as influenza, in young children that have been treated with aspirin (ASA). The major pathological changes occur in the brain and the liver. A noninflammatory cerebral edema develops, leading to increased ICP. Brain function is severely impaired by cerebral edema and the effects of high ammonia levels in serum related to liver dysfunction. The liver enlarges, develops fatty changes in the tissue, and progresses to acute failure. The resultant metabolic abnormalities include hypoglycemia and increased lactic acid in the blood and body fluids, which also contribute to acute encephalopathy. In some cases, the kidneys are also affected.

Injuries

33.
   i. resulting from a mild blow to the head—causes reversible interference with brain function
   ii. bruising of brain tissue with rupture of small blood vessels and edema—usually results from a blunt blow to the head
   iii. simple cracks in the bone
   iv. involves trauma where brain tissue is exposed to the environment
   v. occurs at the base of the skull—often causes leaking of CSF through ears or nose
   vi. occurs when an area of the brain contralateral to the site of direct damage is injured as the brain bounces off the skull

34. (Fig. 14.19)
   i. results from bleeding between the dura and the skull
   ii. between the dura and the arachnoid
   iii. space between the arachnoid and pia mater
   iv. bleeding within the brain

35.
- seizures
- cranial nerve impairment
- otorrhea or rhinorrhea—leaking of CSF from the ear or nose, respectively
- otorrhagia—blood leaking from the ear
- fever due to hypothalamic impairment or cranial or systemic infection
- stress ulcers—from increased gastric secretions

Copyright © 2027 by Elsevier, Inc. All rights reserved, including those for text and data mining, AI training, and similar technologies.

36.
- skull fracture: tissue damage and bleeding resulting in increased ICP, ischemia, and necrosis; compression of brainstem with potential loss of vital functions
- contusion: edema and minor bleeding
- brain motion: tissue damage and bleeding resulting in increased ICP, ischemia, and necrosis; compression of brainstem with potential loss of vital functions
- secondary damage due to bleeding, inflammation, and edema; hematoma and possible infection; tissue damage and bleeding resulting in increased ICP, ischemia, and necrosis; compression of brainstem with potential loss of vital functions
- if unconscious for a prolonged period, other problems may develop; immobility may result in pneumonia or decubitus ulcers

37. (Fig. 14.21)
- hyperextension or hyperflexion of the neck
- dislocation of vertebra
- compression fractures
- penetrating injuries such as stab or bullet wounds
- decreased responses

38. glucocorticoids, antimicrobials, surgery, oxygen therapy

39. (Figs. 14.21, 14.23, and 14.24)
- Damage may be temporary or permanent; laceration of nerve tissue usually results in permanent loss of conduction in affected nerve tracts.
- Complete transection or crushing causes irreversible loss of all function at and below the level of injury.
- Partial transection may allow recovery of some function.
- Bruising is reversible damage when edema and bleeding are mild.
- Prolonged ischemia and necrosis lead to permanent damage.
- Edema and hemorrhage occur above and below the injury.
- Impaired respiration may occur when injury occurs in cervical region.
- Spinal shock can occur.
- Complications include autonomic dysreflexia, immobility, contractures and decubitus ulcers, respiratory and urinary infections, loss of function (e.g., sexual function), and reproductive capacity.

40. (Fig. 14.23) Signs and symptoms depend on the level of the cord at which the injury occurred as well as the time that has elapsed since the injury (*i.e.,* early stage of spinal shock or postspinal shock).

Spinal shock (immediately following injury):
- all function normal above the level of inflammation
- no sensory or motor impulses below the injury
- no reflexes: flaccid paralysis
- no sensation, urinary retention, paralytic ileus
- low, labile blood pressure

Permanent effects—post spinal shock:
- cervical injury—total block:
  - no sensation
  - no voluntary movement (spastic paralysis)
  - no central control of SNS
  - no voluntary control of bladder and bowel
- lumbar injury:
  - normal function upper body
  - no function at level of injury
  - no sensory of voluntary movement below injury
  - reflexes present below injury
  - spastic paralysis
  - bowel and bladder incontinence

41.
- traction or surgery to relieve pressure and repair tissues
- glucocorticoids
- supportive care and rehabilitation to prevent complications related to immobility

42.

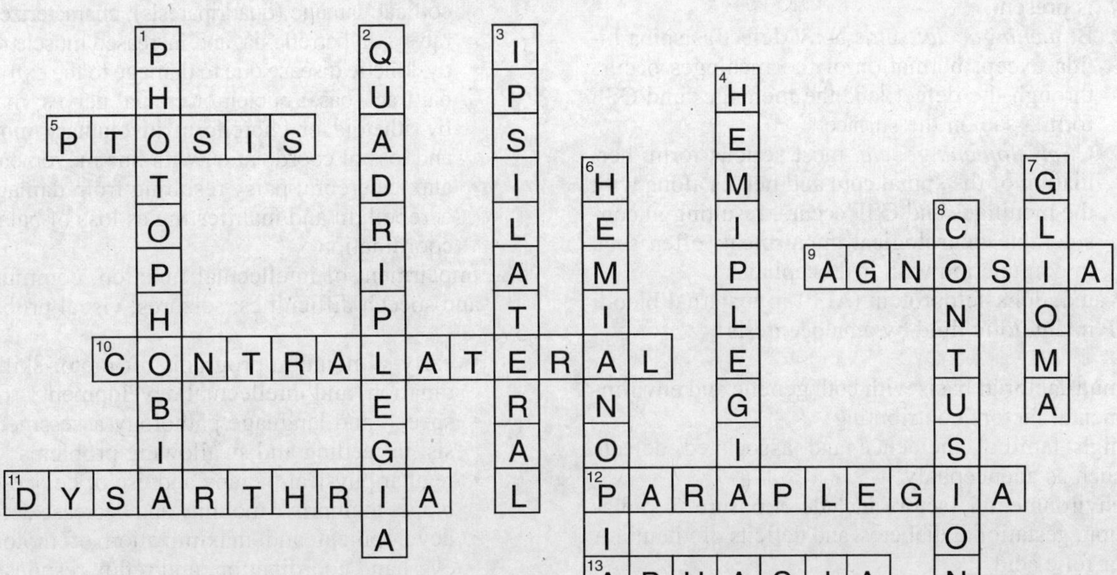

Copyright © 2027 by Elsevier, Inc. All rights are reserved, including those for text and data mining, AI training, and similar technologies.

CONGENITAL NEUROLOGIC DISORDERS

Hydrocephalus

43. a condition in which excess CSF accumulates in the skull, compressing the brain tissue and blood vessels
44. developmental abnormalities such as stenosis or atresia; tumors, infection, or scar tissue at any age
45. Excess CSF leads to compression of brain tissue and blood vessels, which results in brain damage. The amount of brain damage depends on the rate at which pressure increases and the time before treatment.
46. (Fig. 14.25) Noncommunicating, or obstructive, hydrocephalus occurs in babies when the flow of CSF through the ventricular system is blocked. In communicating hydrocephalus, absorption of CSF through subarachnoid villi is impaired, resulting in increased CSF pressure. Infants show head enlargement and developmental delays, while adults experience more severe neurological symptoms due to increased intracranial pressure.
47. It depends on the age of the patient. In neonates or young infants (before suture closure), manifestations include enlarged head, bulging fontanels, dilated scalp veins, eyes showing "sunset" sign, sluggish pupil response, lethargy and restlessness, and shrill cries when infants are picked up. In older children and adults, manifestations include classic signs of increased intracranial pressure.
48. Treatment is surgery to remove the obstruction or provide a shunt for CSF.

Spina Bifida

49. neural tube defect due to failure of the vertebral posterior spinous process to fuse
50. (Fig. 14.26)
    i. A: *spina bifida occulta:* develops when the spinous processes do not fuse, but herniation of the spinal cord and meninges does not occur; may not be visible; often a dimple or tuft of hair is present
    ii. B: *meningocele:* same bony defect as spina bifida except herniation of the meninges occurs through the defect, and the meninges and CSF form a sac on the surface
    iii. C: *myelomeningocele:* most serious form; herniation of the spinal cord and nerves along with the meninges and CSF occurs, resulting in considerable neurological impairment; often seen in conjunction with hydrocephalus
51. elevated alpha-fetoprotein (AFP) in maternal blood; AFP in amniotic fluid by amniocentesis
52.
    - multifactorial basis with both genetic and environmental factors contributing
    - high familial incidence and associated defects such as anencephaly
    - environmental factors include exposure to radiation, gestational diabetes, and deficits of vitamin A or folic acid
53.
    - meningocele and myelomeningocele are visible as protrusions over the spine
    - extent of neurological defect depending on level of the defect (myelomeningocele)
    - impaired sensory and motor function at and below the level of herniation
    - muscle weakness or paralysis
    - fecal and urinary incontinence, depending on the level of damage
54. surgery and occupational and physical therapy to manage the neurological deficits

Cerebral Palsy

55. Major causes of cerebral palsy include hypoxia or ischemia, which can occur prenatally (e.g., due to placental insufficiency or umbilical cord issues), perinatally (e.g., during a difficult delivery causing birth asphyxia), or postnatally (e.g., from vascular occlusion, intracranial hemorrhage, aspiration, or respiratory distress in premature infants). Infections (e.g., maternal rubella or postnatal meningitis) or metabolic abnormalities, such as hypoglycemia in the mother or infant, can also damage the developing brain, leading to cerebral palsy. Additionally, genetic factors or congenital brain malformations may contribute to the condition in some cases. These insults disrupt neural development, causing permanent motor dysfunction characteristic of cerebral palsy.
56. necrosis of brain tissue in the perinatal period as a result of malformation, mechanical trauma, hypoxia, hemorrhage, hypoglycemia, hyperbilirubinemia; necrosis and atrophy may be generalized or localized; all children have some altered mobility and an assortment of other individual problems based on the extent of brain damage
57. (Table 14.9)
    - spastic paralysis due to damage to the pyramidal tracts (diplegia), the motor cortex (hemiparesis), or general cortical damage (quadriparesis); characterized by paralysis, hyperreflexia, and increased muscle tone
    - dyskinetic disease due to damage to the extrapyramidal tract, basal nuclei, or cranial nerves; manifested by athetoid or choreiform involuntary movements and loss of coordination with fine movements
    - ataxic cerebral palsy resulting from damage to the cerebellum and manifesting as loss of balance and coordination
58. impairment of intellectual function; communication and speech difficulties; seizures; visual problems
59.
    - early stimulation programs for motor skills, coordination, and intellectual development
    - speech and language pathology assessment to assist in feeding and swallowing problems
    - regular physical therapy and use of devices such as braces to improve mobility and decrease deformities
    - development and maximization of motor skills, eye-hand coordination, and reflex responses

Copyright © 2027 by Elsevier, Inc. All rights are reserved, including those for text and data mining, AI training, and similar technologies.

- monitoring hearing and vision and appropriate communication therapy
- medications to control seizures

SEIZURE DISORDERS

60. A seizure is an uncontrolled excessive discharge (firing) of neurons in the brain.
61. A seizure results from a sudden spontaneous and uncontrolled depolarization of neurons; it causes abnormal motor and sensory activity and possible loss of consciousness.
62. Primary seizures are idiopathic. Secondary (acquired) seizures have an identifiable cause such as posttraumatic syndrome.
63. initiated by tumor, infection, or hemorrhage in the brain, high fever, and some systemic disorders (renal failure or hypoglycemia) or sudden withdrawal from sedatives or alcohol or narcotics
64. (Box 14.1)
    - *generalized seizure:* has multiple foci in deep structures of both cerebral hemispheres and the brainstem—causes loss of consciousness
    - *partial seizure:* single origin, often in cerebral cortex—may or may not cause altered consciousness
65. An absence or petit mal seizure is a generalized seizure that is more common in children, lasts for 5 to 10 seconds, and may occur many times during the day. There is a brief loss of awareness (child may simply stare into space) and sometimes transient facial movements, which may occur several times a day, with no memory of the episode.
66. In some individuals, signs such as nausea, irritability, depression, or muscle twitching may occur some hours before the onset of a seizure.
67. peculiar visual or auditory or olfactory sensation that immediately precedes the loss of consciousness; examples of auras are the smell of burnt toast, bright flashing lights, buzzing sounds; the significance of an aura is that a seizure is imminent.
68. physical stimuli such as loud noises or bright lights; biochemical stimuli such as stress, excessive premenstrual fluid retention, hypoglycemia, or hyperventilation (alkalosis)
69. A tonic-clonic seizure may occur spontaneously or after simple seizures. The pattern for this type of seizure is:

    tonic stage:
    - nausea, irritability, depression, or muscle twitching
    - aura (which may precede a loss of consciousness in some people)
    - loss of consciousness
    - strong tonic muscle contraction
    - jaws clench, air is forced out of the lungs, a cry escapes, respiration ceases

    clonic stage:
    - muscles contract and relax in a series of jerky movements involving the entire body
    - increased salivation (foaming at the mouth), bowel/bladder incontinence may occur
    - contractions subside, the body turns limp, and consciousness eventually returns
    - person is confused and tired, muscles ache, person falls into deep sleep

    Typical duration is several minutes, should not last longer than 5 minutes.
70. hypoxia, airway obstruction, acidosis, status epilepticus
71. See Emergency Treatment for Seizures box.
72.
    - if individual stops breathing during seizure
    - when a seizure lasts more than 5 minutes
    - when one seizure immediately follows another
    - if individual hurts himself or herself (e.g., due to a fall at onset of seizure)
    - if individual has not recovered consciousness after 30 minutes
73. (Box 14.1)

    simple partial seizure: arises from a single damaged area, often in cortex
    - characterized by repeated motor activity
    - memory and consciousness remain

    complex partial seizure: usually arises from temporal lobe with possible limbic system or frontal lobe involvement
    - characterized by bizarre behavior that may be mistaken for psychiatric condition, such as inappropriate repetitive movements
    - frequently experiences auditory or visual hallucinations
    - individual is unresponsive
74. anticonvulsants and sedatives such as barbiturates
75. Adverse effects of anticonvulsants include leukopenia with increased susceptibility to infection and reduced blood clotting ability and gingival hyperplasia (particularly phenytoin). Adverse effects of barbiturates include increased liver enzyme activity affecting the dosage of other medications, drowsiness, and osteomalacia.
76. Status epilepticus are recurrent tonic-clonic seizures without return to full consciousness. They can be life-threatening. IV diazepam, oxygen, and fluids are used to treat this condition.
77.
    - How well is the individual's disorder controlled—when was the last seizure and how frequently do they occur?
    - Were any known precipitating factors present: stress, bright lights, certain noises or odors, hyperventilation, exercise, hot environmental temperatures, recent alcohol consumption, nitrous oxide?
    - Was there the presence of an "aura", and how much time is there between the aura and the onset of a seizure?
    - How long do seizures usually last?
    - How long does it take to recover from a seizure?
    - What does the individual want you to do if he has a seizure (e.g., who to notify)?
78. awareness and avoidance of potential precipitating factors; stress reduction, which may require sedation (e.g., before a dental treatment)
79. i. EEG; ii MRI

Copyright © 2027 by Elsevier, Inc. All rights are reserved, including those for text and data mining, AI training, and similar technologies.

CHRONIC DEGENERATIVE DISORDERS

Multiple Sclerosis (MS)

80. (Fig. 14.29) progressive demyelinations of neurons in the brain, spinal cord, and cranial nerves
81. unknown etiology; possibly autoimmune disorder with genetic, immunological, and environmental components
82. women between the ages of 20 and 40; individuals of European descent; those living in temperate climates; close relatives of individuals with MS
83. (Fig. 14.29) Plaques are the characteristic lesions of MS and refer to the areas of inflammation and demyelination. These can cause loss of myelin in the white matter of the brain and/or spinal cord which greatly decreases the conductivity of the nerve fibers.
84. motor, sensory, and autonomic
85. There is no definitive test for MS. Multiplicity of effects and recurrences based on patient history and physical examination point to the correct diagnosis. MRIs are best to detect multiple CNS lesions. Often patients have elevated protein, gamma globulin, and lymphocytes in the CSF. Visual evoked potential tests measure the activity of the brain in response to the stimulation of specific sensory pathways and can detect a slowing of conduction due to demyelination. Optical coherence tomography (OCT) is a relatively new imaging tool that can clearly show the retinal structures including the optic and retinal nerves. Since these nerves are often an early target of MS, their condition can give an indication of damage caused by MS.
86. Early manifestations include blurred vision, weakness in the legs, scotoma, diplopia, dysarthria if the cranial nerves are involved, and paresthesias if sensory nerves are affected. Progressive signs are weakness and paralysis extending to upper limbs, loss of coordination and bladder, bowel, and sexual dysfunction. Chronic fatigue and sensory deficits such as paresthesias and loss of position sense in the upper body are also progressive signs. Depression or euphoria may occur later.
87. There is no specific treatment available. The following may be used to control exacerbations:
    - glucocorticoids
    - interferons
    - muscle relaxants
    - avoidance of excessive fatigue, stress, injury, or infection
    - physical therapy and exercise
    - specific therapies for vision, speech, etc.
88. Glucocorticoids will decrease inflammation, and it is possible neural function will return. Interferon will suppress the immune response and may slow progression of the disease.

Parkinson Disease

89. a progressive degenerative disorder affecting motor function
90. There are progressive degenerative changes in the basal nuclei, principally in the substantia nigra. Decreased secretion of dopamine results in an imbalance between excitation and inhibition in the basal nuclei, which causes resting tremors, muscular rigidity, difficulty in initiating movement, and postural instability.
91. (Fig. 14.30) Early manifestations include fatigue, muscle weakness, muscle aching, decreased flexibility, less spontaneous change in facial expression, tremors in the hands at rest, and "pill-rolling" motion. Progressive signs include tremors affecting hands, feet, face, tongue, and lips; increased muscle rigidity, difficulty in initiating movement; bradykinesia and lack of associative involuntary movements; and characteristic stooped posture. Late signs include festination or a propulsive gait; difficulty engaging in complex activities; voice changes; difficulty chewing and swallowing; drooling; mask-like facies; and autonomic dysfunction, such as urinary retention, constipation, and orthostatic hypotension.
92. phenothiazines
93. dopamine; levodopa; selegiline; anticholinergic drugs

ALS, Myasthenia Gravis, and Huntington Disease

94.

	Amyotrophic Lateral Sclerosis (ALS)	Myasthenia Gravis	Huntington Disease
Etiology	Idiopathic, degenerative disorder 10% Genetic	Idiopathic Autoimmune Thymus disorders	Autosomal dominant disorder
Pathophysiology	Progressive loss of neurons in cerebral cortex, brainstem, and spinal cord in diffuse asymmetrical pattern	Development of IgG autoantibodies to acetylcholine receptors, preventing muscle stimulation Facial and ocular muscles first, then arm and trunk	Progressive brain atrophy, especially basal ganglia and frontal cortex Depletion of GABA Decreased brain levels of acetylcholine

Copyright © 2027 by Elsevier, Inc. All rights are reserved, including those for text and data mining, AI training, and similar technologies.

	Amyotrophic Lateral Sclerosis (ALS)	Myasthenia Gravis	Huntington Disease
Manifestations	Loss of fine motor coordination, usually in hands first Stumbling and falls Muscle cramping or twitching Dysarthria Finally, impaired swallowing and respiration	Diplopia; ptosis Loss of facial expression Difficulty chewing and swallowing Marked muscle fatigue and weakness in head, neck, and arms Upper respiratory infections	Rapid, jerky (choreiform) movements in arms and legs Intellectual impairment Progressive rigidity and akinesia, making voluntary movement difficult Progressive dementia
Treatment	No specific treatment Supportive measures Ultimately ventilator	Anticholinesterase agents Glucocorticoids Plasmapheresis to remove antibodies from blood Thymectomy if hyperplastic or if tumor is present	No specific treatment Supportive measures Muscle relaxants to control abnormal movements
Prognosis	Fatal HCO_3^- respiratory failure or infection	Fatal HCO_3^- respiratory failure or infection	Incurable—progressive Detection of carriers and genetic counseling

DEMENTIA

95. Alzheimer disease; cerebrovascular disease-multiple microinfarcts; Creutzfeldt-Jakob disease; AIDS
96.
    - progressive cortical atrophy—leads to dilated ventricles and widening of sulci
    - neurofibrillary tangles in the neurons and senile plaques containing beta-amyloid precursor protein
    - deficit in neurotransmitter acetylcholine
97. A specific cause is unknown; at least four defective genes on different chromosomes have been associated with the disease.
98. In the early stage, manifestations include gradual loss of memory and lack of concentration and an impaired ability to learn new information and to reason. There are behavioral changes such as irritability and hostility. Cognitive function, memory, and language skills decline; apathy, indifference, and confusion become marked; managing activities of daily living becomes increasingly difficult. In the later stages, there is an inability to recognize family members; lack of awareness or interest in environment; incontinence, and loss of functionality.

MENTAL DISORDERS

99. The following types of behavior may be exhibited:
    - positive symptoms such as delusions and bizarre behavior
    - negative symptoms such as flat emotions and decreased speech
    - disorganized thought processes
    - delusions of false beliefs and ideas such as grandeur or power over others
    - poor problem-solving ability
    - short attention span
    - impaired communication
    - hallucinations or abnormal sensory perception
    - social withdrawal
    - personal self-care neglected
100. frequently cause side effects related to excessive extrapyramidal activity (or parkinsonian signs) such as dystonia and tardive dyskinesia: involuntary muscle spasms in the face, neck, arms, or legs
101.
    - selective serotonin reuptake inhibitors (SSRIs) such as Prozac
    - serotonin-norepinephrine reuptake inhibitors (SNRIs) such as Effexor
    - tricyclic antidepressants (TCAs) such as Elavil
    - monamine oxidase (MAO) inhibitors such as Parnate

Panic Disorder

102. repeated episodes of intense fear without provocation, palpitations or tachycardia, hyperventilation, sweating, sensation of choking or smothering, nausea

SPINAL CORD DISORDER

Herniated Disk

103. (Fig. 14.33) protrusion of the nucleus pulposus (the inner gelatinous component of the intervertebral disk) through a tear in the annulus fibrosus, the outer covering of the intervertebral disc
104. If pressure on the nerve tissue or blood supply is prolonged or severe, permanent nerve damage might occur.
105. The most common site of a herniated disc is at the lumbosacral discs, at L4 to L5 or L5 to S1. This

Copyright © 2027 by Elsevier, Inc. All rights are reserved,
including those for text and data mining, AI training, and similar technologies.

results in lower back pain, radiating down one or both legs, that is exacerbated by coughing or straight leg raising. Paresthesia or numbness and tingling, as well as muscle weakness, if compression is severe (motor nerves), may result.

106. conservative treatment, including bed rest; application of heat, ice, or traction, or drugs such as analgesics, antiinflammatory agents, and skeletal muscle relaxants; surgery if compression persists: laminectomy or discectomy; chemonucleolysis; fusion

CONSOLIDATION

107.
- nature of the disorder—etiology, is it progressive?
- duration and degree of impairment
- Who is the primary care provider?

108.
- Try to arrange for person who is responsible for care to be present at appointments.
- Always provide written instructions regarding follow-up treatment, etc.—this is particularly important for individuals who are living in group homes or nursing homes where there are multiple care providers.
- Provide clear explanations.
- Provide demonstrations whenever possible (e.g., how to floss teeth).

109.
i. multiple sclerosis
ii. myasthenia gravis
iii. Parkinson and Huntington
iv. Alzheimer
v. Parkinson
vi. Huntington
vii. amyotrophic lateral sclerosis
viii. Huntington
ix. multiple sclerosis, myasthenia gravis
x. Parkinson
xi. multiple sclerosis, Alzheimer
xii. Huntington and Alzheimer
xiii. Parkinson
xiv. Alzheimer
xv. Creutzfeldt-Jakob disease

CHAPTER 15: Disorders of the Eye, Ear, and Other Sensory Organs

EYE

1. See Fig. 15.1 of the text.
A. Medial rectus muscle, B. Retinal artery, C. Retinal vein, D. Optic nerve, E. Central retinal artery and vein, F. Meninges, G. Optic disc, H. Fovea centralis, I. Sclera, J. Choroid, K. Retina, L. Lateral rectus muscle, M. Conjunctiva, N. Posterior chamber, O. Anterior chamber, P. Lens, Q. Cornea, R. Pupil, S. Iris, T. Canal of Schlemm, U. Ciliary muscle, V. Suspensory ligament, W. Posterior cavity

2.
i. measures visual acuity
ii. checks central and peripheral vision
iii. assesses interocular pressure
iv. examines interior eye structures
v. measures the angle of the anterior chamber

3.
i. nearsightedness
ii. farsightedness
iii. farsightedness associated with aging
iv. irregular curvature in the cornea or lens
v. double vision or paralysis of upper eyelid

4.
i. infection involving a hair follicle on the eyelid—usually caused by staphylococci
ii. inflammation or infection involving the conjunctiva: inflammation can be caused by allergies or irritating chemicals; infection can be caused by *Staphylococcus aureus* (pinkeye); *Chlamydia trachomatis* and gonorrhea cause infections of the respiratory tract and may infect eyes of newborns; *Neisseria gonorrhea* can cause infection by self-inoculation
iii. eye infection caused by *Chlamydia trachomatis*—causes follicles to develop on the inner surface of eyelids
iv. infected cornea, very painful, can be caused by the Herpes simplex virus

5. (Fig. 15.4) increased intraocular pressure caused by an excessive accumulation of aqueous humor
6. (Fig. 15.4) Narrow-angle glaucoma occurs when the angle between the cornea and the iris in the anterior chamber is decreased by factors such as abnormal anterior insertion of the iris. Wide-angle, or chronic, glaucoma is a degenerative disorder in older people. The trabecular network and canal of Schlemm become obstructed, diminishing the outflow of aqueous humor.
7. the elderly, older than 50
8.
- increased intraocular pressure
- loss of peripheral vision
- corneal edema and altered light refraction, leading to blurred vision and appearance of "halos" around lights
- mild eye discomfort
- acute episodes may be triggered by pupil dilation (narrow-angle)
- eye pain, nausea, and headache; blurred vision; bulging and cloudy cornea
- pupil dilated and unresponsive to light

9. Therapeutic interventions include regular administration of β-adrenergic blockers (reduce secretions) or cholinergic agents (contract the pupil) and/or surgery, such as laser iridotomy, for acute narrow-angle glaucoma if severe.

Copyright © 2027 by Elsevier, Inc. All rights are reserved, including those for text and data mining, AI training, and similar technologies.

10.

	Cataract	Macular Degeneration	Retinal Detachment
Etiology	Aging, trauma, or congenital factors Metabolic abnormalities Maternal infections	Aging Genetics Environmental factors	Marked myopia Aging
Pathology	Progressive clouding of lens	Growth of membrane over retina, starting at fovea centralis	Retina lifted from choroid as vitreous seeps behind tear, retinal cells stop functioning and may die
Effect on vision	Progressive blurring and darkening of vision	Loss of central vision Altered depth perception	"Floaters"—light or dark floating spots Growing area of blackness in visual field
Treatment	Lens removal and replacement with intraocular lens	Limited by type Photoactivated drugs Laser treatment	Scleral buckling Laser therapy

11. For the dry type of age-related macular degeneration (AMD), nutrition is assessed to ensure that vitamin, mineral, and antioxidant intake are sufficient. A high-dose formulation of antioxidants and zinc has been shown to reduce the risk. In the wet type of AMD, photodynamic therapy (photosensitive drug plus laser) may help seal off neovasculature. The older method, laser photocoagulation may also be used to seal vessels without the photo-activated drug, Visudyne, which is used in photodynamic therapy. The new drug, pegaptanib (Macugen) may slow vascular growth, and therapy using the drug anti-vascular endothelial growth factor has shown promise. An intraocular injection of this medication inhibits the formation of new blood vessels behind the retina and may keep the retina free of leakage.
12.
    i. cataracts
    ii. macular degeneration
    iii. glaucoma
    iv. macular degeneration
    v. glaucoma
    vi. glaucoma

EAR

13. See Fig. 15.8 of the text.
    A. Temporal bone, B. Auditory ossicles, C. Malleus, D. Incus, E. Stapes, F. Semicircular canals, G. Oval window, H. Vestibular nerve, I. Cochlear nerve, J. Auditory nerve (VIII), K. Cochlea containing organ of Corti, L. Vestibule, M. Auditory (eustachian) tube, N. Inner ear, O. Middle ear, P. External ear, Q. Tympanic membrane, R. External auditory canal, S. Pinna
14. Conduction deafness occurs when sound is blocked in the external or middle ear. For example, wax accumulation, a foreign object, scar tissue, or adhesions may cause conduction deafness. Sensorineural deafness is due to damage to the organ of Corti or auditory nerve. For example, infection, particularly viral, such as rubella, influenza, or herpes; head trauma; or ototoxic drugs may cause sensorineural deafness.
15. Otitis media is an inflammation or infection of the middle ear cavity. Common causative bacteria include *Haemophilus influenzae,* pneumococci, β-hemolytic streptococci, and staphylococci. Viruses can also cause otitis media—viral infections are often followed by a secondary bacterial infection.
16. Antibacterials if caused by bacteria; ibuprofen or acetaminophen if it is a viral infection—to reduce discomfort; viral infection can be followed by antibacterials if infection does not clear up.
17. Otitis externa is an infection of the external auditory canal and the pinna. It is usually bacterial but may be fungal as well.
18. a disorder of the inner ear or labyrinth due to intermittent development of excessive endolymph that stretches the membranes and interferes with function of the hair cells in the cochlea and vestibule; manifestations include episodes lasting minutes or hours causing vertigo, tinnitus, and unilateral hearing loss
19.
    i. infants and young children
    ii. swimmers; frequent users of ear plugs or earphones
    iii. beginning in adults between 30 and 50 years of age

CHAPTER 16: Endocrine System Disorders

1. See Fig. 16.1 of the text.
    A. Pituitary gland, B. Pineal gland, C. Four parathyroid glands on posterior thyroid, D. Thyroid gland, E. Thymus, F. Adrenal gland, G. Pancreas, H. Kidney, I. Ovary in female, J. Testis in male

Copyright © 2027 by Elsevier, Inc. All rights are reserved, including those for text and data mining, AI training, and similar technologies.

2. Hormones are chemical messengers and can be classified by:
   - *Action:* control or hormone levels, *i.e.,* blood calcium levels
   - *Source:* endocrine organ, *i.e.,* adrenal gland
   - *Chemical structure:* amino acid derivatives or steroids
3. negative feedback
4. an excessive amount of hormone or a hormonal deficit
5. radioimmunoassay and immunochemical assays

DIABETES MELLITUS

6. (Table 16.2) familial history (type 1); obesity, advancing age (type 2)
7. (Table 16.2)
   - *Type 1:* genetic factor (family history); autoimmune destruction of pancreatic beta cells
   - *Type 2:* familial, lifestyle, and environmental factors, especially obesity
8. An insulin deficit leads to the following sequence of events and can be categorized into the initial stage and progressive effects:
   Initial stage:
   - decreased transportation and use of glucose
   - hyperglycemia
   - glucosuria
   - polyuria with loss of fluid and electrolytes
   - fluid loss through the urine and high blood glucose levels—dehydration
   - polydipsia due to dehydration
   - lack of nutrients entering the cells, stimulating appetite and leading to polyphagia

   Progressive effects:
   - catabolism of fats and proteins due to lack of glucose in cells; resulting in ketosis as metabolites accumulate—ketoacidosis
   - ketonuria
   - glomerular filtration drops, resulting in decompensated metabolic acidosis
9. (Fig. 16.4) The lack of glucose in cells results in catabolism of fats, leading to excessive buildup of fatty acids and their metabolites, ketone (ketoacids).
10. (Table 16.3) Warning signs include:
    - *polyuria:* hyperglycemia results in excess glucose in the urine as renal tubular reabsorption capacity is exceeded; the glucose in the filtrate exerts osmotic pressure, increasing the volume of urine produced
    - *polydipsia:* fluid and electrolyte loss due to glucosuria results in dehydration and stimulation of the thirst response (hypothalamus)
    - *polyphagia:* lack of nutrients in cells stimulates appetite
    - *weight loss:* particularly with type 1, due to fat catabolism
11. Diagnosis is established from the following: fasting blood glucose level, glucose tolerance test, and glycosylated hemoglobin test.
12. Dietary modifications include dieting to reduce weight or maintain optimum weight; adding more complex carbohydrates, getting adequate protein, and taking in low saturated fats and fiber to reduce cholesterol levels; having minimal intake of simple and refined sugars; and balancing and reducing food intake to match insulin availability, metabolic needs, and activity level.
13. Oral hypoglycemics act in a number of different ways to lower blood sugar; some stimulate beta cells to release more insulin, others reduce insulin resistance of cells and hepatic glucose production, and another type increases cell sensitivity to insulin.
14.
    - hypoglycemia
    - gastrointestinal disturbances; anorexia, nausea, vomiting
    - anemia
    - pruritus (itching)
    - liver and kidney damage
    - metallic taste (with metformin)
15. The various forms of insulin differ in onset of action, peak insulin levels, and duration of action.
16. Insulin can be administered by subcutaneous injections, continuous subcutaneous infusion ("insulin pump"), or inhalation, which was just approved by the U.S. Food and Drug Administration.
17. (Fig. 16.3) Factors that could precipitate a hypoglycemic or insulin reaction include increased physical exercise, skipping a meal or fasting, delayed or inadequate food intake, insulin overdose (too much insulin), and nutritional and/or fluid and electrolyte imbalances due to nausea and vomiting.
18. Verify that patients have eaten and taken appropriate medications.
    Schedule appointments that do not unduly delay meals.
19. See Table 16.4.
20. Diabetic neuropathy is a disorder of peripheral nerves that produces impaired sensation, numbness, tingling, weakness, and muscle wasting. It results from ischemia and changes in the metabolic process. Degenerative changes occur in both unmyelinated and myelinated fibers. There is a risk of tissue trauma and infection. Autonomic nerve degeneration leads to bladder incontinence, impotence, diarrhea, and impaired vasomotor reflexes. Vascular impairment decreases tissue resistance and slows healing; sensory impairment means that an individual may not realize that he has injured himself and therefore does not implement appropriate measures.
21. Risk of infection is greatly increased when vascular and sensory impairment coexist.
22.
    - tuberculosis
    - infections in the feet and hands
    - fungal infections
    - urinary tract infections
    - periodontal disease
23. There may be delayed healing because of decreased circulation to the injured site due to both macroangiopathy and microangiopathy. Individuals are more prone to infections, which will further delay healing.
24. (Chapter 22) diabetes that develops during pregnancy and usually ends with the delivery of the infant

Copyright © 2027 by Elsevier, Inc. All rights are reserved, including those for text and data mining, AI training, and similar technologies.

25. (Figs. 16.3 and 16.4)

	Hypoglycemic Shock	Ketoacidosis
Other names	Insulin shock Insulin reaction	Diabetic coma
Cause	Hypoglycemia	Hyperglycemia
Precipitating factors	Increased physical exercise Skipping a meal or fasting Delayed or inadequate food intake Insulin overdose—too much insulin Nutritional and/or fluid and electrolyte imbalances due to nausea and vomiting	Excessive food and/or alcohol intake Inadequate insulin—skipped or delayed Increased requirement for insulin: infection, stress, glucocorticoids
Speed of onset	Rapid	Slow
Manifestations	Apprehensive, headache Pale, cold, diaphoretic, "clammy" Hungry, thirsty Appears intoxicated: unexpected behavior, slurred speech, incoherent, disoriented, staggering gait Difficulty problem solving Muscle twitching, tremors Seizures Permanent brain damage Death	Increased hunger and thirst Polyuria Fatigue, confusion Nausea and vomiting Signs of dehydration: flushed, warm, dry skin and mucous membranes Acetone breath Tachycardia and lowered blood pressure Rapid, deep breathing Loss of consciousness
Emergency treatment	Glucose in rapidly absorbed form	Insulin Fluid and electrolyte replacement Sodium bicarbonate
Speed of response to emergency treatment	Rapid	Slow
Prevention	Never interfere with normal mealtimes of a diabetic Never tell a diabetic to fast without seeking medical consult Have available a ready source of glucose Careful observation for warning signs	Never tell a diabetic not to take medication without medical consult Careful observation for warning signs

26.

	Type 1 (IDDM)	Type 2 (NIDDM)
Percentage of individuals with DM	10%	90%
Age at onset	Preadolescent	Older than 30
Speed of onset of symptoms	Acute	Insidious
Family history	Yes	Very strong
Body build (BMI)	Thin	Obese
Presence of autoantibodies	Yes	No
Insulin receptor defects	No	Yes
Severity of manifestations	Acute	Mild
Stability (*i.e.,* maintenance of normal blood glucose)	More difficult	More stable

Copyright © 2027 by Elsevier, Inc. All rights are reserved, including those for text and data mining, AI training, and similar technologies.

	Type 1 (IDDM)	Type 2 (NIDDM)
Frequency of complications	Frequent	Less common
Occurrence of ketoacidosis	Frequent	Less common
Frequency of hypoglycemia	Frequent	Less common
Treatment with insulin	Always	Less common
Treatment with oral hypoglycemics	No	Frequent

BMI, body mass index; *DM,* diabetes mellitus; *IDDM,* insulin-dependent diabetes mellitus; *NIDDM,* non–insulin-dependent diabetes mellitus.

PARATHYROID DISORDERS

27.
- *Hypoparathyroidism:* congenital lack of parathyroid glands, following surgery or radiation in the neck region, or as a result of autoimmune disease
- *Hyperparathyroidism:* adenoma, hyperplasia, secondary to renal failure

28. (Fig. 16.11) Hypoparathyroidism leads to hypocalcemia, which affects nerve and muscle function. It can lead to weak cardiac muscle contractions but increased excitability of nerves, leading to spontaneous contractions of skeletal muscle: twitching and spasms.
29. (Fig. 16.11) Hyperparathyroidism causes hypercalcemia, which leads to forceful cardiac contractions; osteoporosis due to excess bone demineralization; and increased predisposition to kidney stones.

ACROMEGALY

30. excess growth hormone secretions from a pituitary adenoma in the adult
31. (Fig. 16.12)
Manifestations include:
- bones that become broader and heavier
- soft tissues that grow, resulting in enlarged hands and feet
- a thicker skull
- changes in facial features

Complications include:
- nerve and blood vessel compression in the skull
- carpal tunnel syndrome
- arthritis
- diabetes
- hypertension and cardiovascular disease

ANTIDIURETIC HORMONE

32. Diabetes insipidus is due to insufficient antidiuretic hormone (ADH; also known as vasopressin) release—no sugar in urine; diabetes mellitus is caused by a lack or insufficient release of insulin or insulin resistance—sugar in urine.

THYROID DISORDERS

33. (Figs. 16.13 and 16.14) A goiter is an enlargement of the thyroid gland that is often visible on the neck; it is caused by hypothyroidism (endemic goiter) and hyperthyroidism (toxic goiter).
34. (Table 16.5)

	Hyperthyroidism	Hypothyroidism
Forms	Graves disease Adult: myxedema	Infant: cretinism
Etiology	Autoimmune: thyroid-stimulating antibodies Adenoma: thyroid or pituitary Toxic goiter	Congenital: • Thyroid agenesis or dysgenesis • Lower TSH or T3 and T4 Adult: • Autoimmune (Hashimoto's disease) • Surgical removal • Drugs
Serum T3 and T4 levels	High	Low
Metabolic rate	High	Low

Copyright © 2027 by Elsevier, Inc. All rights are reserved, including those for text and data mining, AI training, and similar technologies.

	Hyperthyroidism	Hypothyroidism
Nervous system effects	Restlessness, anxiety, irritability Insomnia Tremors Impaired concentration	Child: severe mental retardation Decreased reflexes Fatigue, sluggishness Headache Slow intellectual functions Coma
Cardiovascular effects	Tachycardia Palpitations, arrhythmias Increased blood pressure Cardiomegaly Severe: angina pectoris, myocardial infarction	Bradycardia Decreased cardiac output Decreased blood pressure
Respiratory effects	Hyperventilation Dyspnea	Hypoventilation
Skeletal effects	Increased resorption Advanced bone age Osteoporosis	Retarded bone age "Stubby hands"
Muscular effects	Increased tone leading to tremors and twitching Diarrhea	Decreased tone and reflexes Muscle weakness Decreased peristalsis leading to constipation, flatulence, and abdominal distention
Skin and hair	Increased sweating Flushed warm skin Soft nails Thin, silky hair	Pale; yellowish hue Cool Dry and rough Hair brittle and coarse Alopecia Loss of lateral third of eyebrows
Temperature tolerance	Increased body temperature Heat intolerance	Decreased body temperature Cold intolerance
Eyes	Exophthalmos Decreased blinking and eye movements "Lid lag"	Puffy
Body weight	Decreased with increased appetite	Increased with decreased appetite
Presence of goiter	With Graves disease	With endemic goiter
Treatment	Antithyroid agents Radioactive iodine Thyroidectomy	Replacement therapy

TSH, thyroid-stimulating hormone

ADRENAL DISORDERS

35. (Figs. 16.16 to 16.18; Table 16.6)

	Cushing Syndrome	Addison Disease
Etiology	Adrenal tumor Glucocorticoids therapy Pituitary tumor Paraneoplastic syndrome	Autoimmune destruction Prolonged treatment with corticosteroids Infections: tuberculosis, fungi, cancer

Copyright © 2027 by Elsevier, Inc. All rights are reserved, including those for text and data mining, AI training, and similar technologies.

	Cushing Syndrome	Addison Disease
Physical appearance	Round "moon face" Thinning of skin Purple striae Ecchymoses Cervical or supraclavicular fat pads—"buffalo hump" Hirsutism Alopecia Protruding abdomen	Hyperpigmentation of skin, particularly in creases—also buccal mucosa and tongue—"bronzing"
Fluid and electrolytes	Increased Na^+ and Cl^- Decreased K^+ Increased HCO_3^- and decreased H^+ Water retention resulting in edema	Decreased Na^+ and Cl^- Increased K^+ Increased H^+ and decreased HCO_3^- Dehydration
Blood pressure	Increased	Decreased
Blood sugar	Increased	Normal or decreased
Musculoskeletal effects	Atrophy Osteoporosis	Weakness
Inflammatory response	Decreased	Decreased
Immune response	Decreased	Decreased
Response to stress	Decreased	Decreased
Treatment	Surgery Palliative treatment: diuretics, antihypertensives, hypoglycemics or insulin antibiotics, etc.	Replacement therapy

36. Excessive glucocorticoids depress both inflammation and immunity, thereby impairing normal defenses. Antibacterial drugs are prescribed to prevent infection.

MULTIPLE ENDOCRINE NEOPLASIA TYPE I

37. Multiple Endocrine Neoplasia Type 1 (MEN1) causes tumors to develop in the parathyroid glands, the pituitary gland, the pancreas as well as sites in the digestive tract such as the stomach and the duodenum. MEN1 can also cause benign tumors in other endocrine glands as well as other tissues including the adrenal glands, the lungs, the meninges and the skin. Multiple tumors will often appear in different tissues at the same time.

CONSOLIDATION

38.
- i. thyroid (T3 and T4) hypersecretion
- ii. growth hormone hypersecretion as a child
- iii. hyposecretion of thyroid hormones T3 and T4 as an adult
- iv. hyposecretion of ADH
- v. growth hormone hypersecretion as an adult
- vi. hypersecretion of glucocorticoids
- vii. hyposecretion of growth hormone
- viii. hyposecretion of insulin
- ix. hyposecretion of mineralocorticoids, glucocorticoids, and androgens
- x. hyposecretion of thyroid hormones as a child

39.
- i. diabetes mellitus, Cushing, acromegaly
- ii. hyperthyroidism
- iii. diabetes mellitus, Addison, Cushing
- iv. hypothyroidism
- v. Cushing hyperthyroidism, hyperparathyroidism
- vi. cretinism (hypothyroidism as child)
- vii. hyperparathyroidism
- viii. Addison, hypothyroidism
- ix. hypothyroidism—cretinism, hyposecretion of growth hormone
- x. Addison
- xi. diabetes mellitus type 1, hyperthyroidism—Graves, hypothyroidism—Hashimoto
- xii. inappropriate ADH syndrome, hypothyroidism—myxedema, Cushing
- xiii. hyperthyroidism—Graves
- xiv. hypothyroidism
- xv. Cushing
- xvi. Cushing, hypothyroidism

Copyright © 2027 by Elsevier, Inc. All rights are reserved, including those for text and data mining, AI training, and similar technologies.

xvii. Addison, Cushing, hyperthyroidism
xviii. diabetes mellitus, inappropriate ADH syndrome, hyperthyroidism, Cushing
xix. diabetes mellitus, hyperthyroidism
xx. hyperthyroidism (Graves), hypothyroidism (endemic)
xxi. acromegaly
xxii. hyperthyroidism
xxiii. inappropriate ADH syndrome, Addison
xxiv. hypoparathyroidism

CHAPTER 17: Digestive System Disorders

1. See Fig. 17.1 of the text.
   A. Parotid salivary gland, B. Oropharynx, C. Submandibular salivary gland, D. Diaphragm, E. Cardiac sphincter, F. Stomach, G. Pyloric sphincter, H. Pancreas, I. Transverse colon, J. Descending colon, K. Jejunum, L. Sigmoid colon, M. Rectum, N. Anus, O. Appendix, P. Cecum, Q. Ileum, R. Ileocecal valve, S. Ascending colon, T. Large intestine, U. Duodenal papilla, V. Duodenum, W. Common bile duct, X. Gallbladder, Y. Liver, Z. Esophagus, AA. Trachea, BB. Sublingual salivary gland, CC. Tooth, DD. Tongue, EE. Mouth, FF. Hard palate
2.
   a) drug used to decrease nausea and vomiting; iv. antiemetic
   b) formation of gallstones; x. cholelithiasis
   c) greasy, loose stools; i. steatorrhea
   d) loss of appetite; v. anorexia
   e) opportunistic oral fungal infection; viii. candidiasis
   f) outpouching of the mucosa in colon; xi. diverticulum
   g) tarry stools caused by bleeding; ii. melena
   h) difficulty swallowing; iii. dysphagia
   i) inflammation of tissue surrounding the teeth; ix. gingivitis
   j) retention of feces; vii. impaction
   k) vomit containing blood; vi. hematemesis
3.
   - distention or irritation in digestive tract: distention due to gas following abdominal surgery; constipation
   - unpleasant sights or smells: sight of blood; odor of emesis or feces
   - pain or stress: performance anxiety; after surgery; going to dentist
   - stimulation of vestibular apparatus in inner ear: motion sickness; amusement rides
   - increased intracranial pressure: brain tumors, hydrocephalus; cerebral hemorrhage
   - stimulation of chemoreceptor trigger zone: drugs, alcohol
4. (Table 17.3)
   - treat cause (e.g., analgesics for pain, laxatives or enema to relieve constipation)
   - antiemetic drugs
   - sedatives
   - antacids
   - good ventilation to remove noxious odors
5.
   - increased age and weakness of smooth muscles in the intestines
   - inadequate dietary fiber
   - inadequate fluid intake
   - failure to respond to the defecation reflex
   - muscle weakness and inactivity
   - neurological disorders such as multiple sclerosis and spinal cord trauma
   - drugs, such as opiates, CNS depressants, or anticholinergic drugs
   - some antacids, iron medications, and bulk laxatives (with insufficient fluid intake)
   - obstruction caused by tumors or strictures
6. increased fiber and fluid intake
7. (Fig. 17.11) Causes include:
   - A: esophageal fibrosis
   - B: esophageal compression
   - C: esophageal diverticulum
   - D: congenital atresia of the esophagus
   - E: congenital tracheoesophageal fistula
   - F: neurological damage to cranial nerves V, VII, IX, X, and XII
   - G: achalasia
8. (Fig. 17.13) Part of the stomach is elevated and protrudes through an opening (hiatus) in the diaphragm into the thoracic cavity.
9. Signs and symptoms include postprandial heartburn or pyrosis, a brief substernal burning sensation, often accompanied by sour taste; belching from regurgitation of gastric contents, especially when in a reclining position; and dysphagia.
10. eliminating factors that reduce lower esophageal sphincter (LES) pressure, such as caffeine, fatty foods, alcohol, cigarette smoking, and certain drugs
11. GERD is gastroesophageal reflux disease, the periodic flow of gastric contents into the esophagus. GERD is caused by hiatal hernia as well as other conditions that lower LES pressure or increase intraabdominal pressure.
12. (Table 17.3) antacids; histamine2 (H2 receptor) antagonist agents; proton pump inhibitors
13. Acute gastritis is an inflammation of the gastric mucosa due to a variety of causes, including infection, food or drug allergy, ingestion of spicy or irritating food, excessive alcohol intake, ingestion of aspirin or other ulcerogenic drugs, ingestion of toxic substances, radiation, or chemotherapy. Acute gastroenteritis is inflammation of both the stomach and intestine, usually caused by infection but may result from food or drug allergies.
14.

	Acute Gastritis	**Chronic Gastritis**
Etiology	Infections	Peptic ulcers
	Food allergies	Alcohol abuse
	Spicy or irritating foods	Aging

Copyright © 2027 by Elsevier, Inc. All rights are reserved, including those for text and data mining, AI training, and similar technologies.

	Acute Gastritis	Chronic Gastritis
	Drugs: aspirin; chemotherapy	Pernicious anemia
	Ingestion of corrosive or toxic substances	
	Radiation	
Signs and symptoms	Epigastric discomfort	Anorexia, nausea, vomiting
	Epigastric pain; cramps	
	Intolerance of spicy foods	
	Hematemesis	

15. See Table 17.4.
16. Enterotoxigenic *E. coli* (ETEC) causes diarrhea in infants and travelers in countries in which proper sanitation is lacking. Organism colonizes the small intestine and produces enterotoxins that may cause minor discomfort to severe cholera-like symptoms.
    Enteroinvasive *E. coli* (EIEC) penetrates and reproduces in and destroys the epithelial cells of the colon. The organism does not produce enterotoxins but causes severe diarrhea and fever.
    Enteropathogenic *E. coli* (EPEC) is very similar to EIEC; however, it is reported to produce an enterotoxin similar to *Shigella.*
    Enteroaggregative *E. coli* (EAggEC) produces persistent diarrhea in young children. In addition to producing an enteroaggregative heat stabile toxin, it also produces a hemolysin produced by strains that commonly cause urinary tract infections.
    Enterohemorrhagic *E. coli* (EHEC) is caused by a specific strain O157:H7. These strains of *E. coli* release verocytotoxins (*Shigella*-like toxins) in the intestine, which cause damage to the mucosa and blood vessel walls, and subsequently may affect blood vessels in the kidneys and elsewhere.

ULCERS

17. (Fig. 17.14) Ulcers occur in the proximal duodenum (most common), antrum of the stomach, and lower esophagus.
18. Factors include decreased mucosal resistance (gastric ulcers), excessive HCl or pepsin secretion (duodenal ulcers), and presence of bacterium *H. pylori.*
19. Acid or pepsin penetrates the mucosal barrier. Tissues are exposed to continued damage because of acid diffusion into the gastric wall. Ulcers may erode more deeply into muscle layers and eventually perforate the wall. Inflammation surrounds the crater. Bleeding occurs when erosion invades a blood vessel. Bleeding may involve persistent loss of small amounts of blood or massive hemorrhage, depending on the size of the blood vessel involved.
20. Complications include:
    - hemorrhage
    - perforation, resulting in chemical peritonitis and, ultimately, bacterial peritonitis
    - obstruction of the digestive tract due to scarring and stricture formation
21. Signs and symptoms include:
    - epigastric burning or aching pain, usually 2 to 3 hours after meals and at night
    - heartburn, nausea, vomiting, and weight loss, especially after alcohol or irritating food
    - iron deficiency anemia or occult blood in the stool
22. Treatments include:
    - drug therapy: usually combination of antimicrobials and acid reducers; coating agents or antacids for symptomatic relief
    - reducing exacerbating factors
    - vagotomy
    - partial gastrectomy or pyloroplasty in patients with perforated or bleeding ulcers

CANCER

23.

	Etiology	Pathophysiology	Symptoms and Complications	Treatment
Esophagus	Chronic esophagitis Hiatal hernia Alcohol abuse Smoking	Circumferential or mass causing obstruction	Dysphagia	Surgery and radiation
Stomach	Diet: nitrates and smoked foods Genetics Chronic atrophic gastritis Polyps	Ulcerative-type lesion in mucosa or protruding mass or polyp Infiltrates into muscularis and serosa Spreads to liver and ovaries	Asymptomatic until late Indigestion Feelings of fullness Weight loss and fatigue Occult blood in stool Iron deficiency anemia	Combination therapy: surgery (gastric resection), chemotherapy, and radiation

Copyright © 2027 by Elsevier, Inc. All rights reserved, including those for text and data mining, AI training, and similar technologies.

	Etiology	Pathophysiology	Symptoms and Complications	Treatment
Liver	Cirrhosis Hepatitis B and C Prolonged exposure to carcinogenic chemicals Metastases from abdominal organs	A mass that obstructs bile ducts and hepatic sinusoids Frequent site of metastases from other sites	Anorexia, vomiting, weight loss Jaundice Portal hypertension Splenomegaly	Chemotherapy Resection if tumor is single and not large
Pancreas	Cigarette smoking Genetics	Mass that obstructs ducts Congestion and inflammation Pancreatitis Early metastases	Abdominal pain Weight loss Jaundice	Surgery, radiation, and chemotherapy
Colorectal	Age: over 55 Familial multiple polyposis Ulcerative colitis	May be polypoid May be ulcerative If circumferential, may cause obstruction Metastasize to liver	Cramping Feeling of incomplete emptying Change in bowel pattern and fecal consistency Occult blood in stool or melena	Surgery, both curative and palliative; may be accompanied by radiation and chemotherapy

GALLBLADDER DISEASE

24. women with high cholesterol levels in the bile; obesity, high cholesterol intake, and multiparity; use of oral contraceptives or estrogen supplements; individuals with hemolytic anemia, alcoholic cirrhosis, or biliary tract infections
25. Signs and symptoms include sudden severe waves of pain in the upper right quadrant of the abdomen or epigastric area, often radiating to the back or right shoulder; nausea and vomiting; increasing and then decreasing pain (if the stone moves on); and increasing pain followed by jaundice.

LIVER DISEASE

26. (Fig. 17.20)
    - prehepatic; results from excessive destruction of red blood cells (RBCs) (e.g., physiological jaundice of some newborns, hemolytic anemias, transfusion reactions)
    - intrahepatic: due to liver disease resulting in impaired uptake of bilirubin from the blood and decreased bilirubin conjugation (e.g., individuals with liver disease such as hepatitis or cirrhosis)
    - posthepatic: obstruction of biliary flow due to congenital atresia of the bile ducts, cholelithiasis; inflammation or tumors of the liver
27. infectious mononucleosis or amebiasis; chemical or drug toxicity

28. (Table 17.5)

	Hepatitis A	Hepatitis B	Hepatitis C
Causative agent	HAV: RNA virus	HBV: double-stranded DNA virus	HCV: RNA virus
Transmission	Oral-fecal: "enteric"	Blood and body fluids	Blood and body fluids
High-risk groups	Individuals living in large institutions (e.g., prisons, nursing homes) Children with poor toileting behavior People living with inadequate sanitation and water for hygiene Travelers to developing countries Individuals who engage in oral/anal sex	IV drug users Individuals engaging in unprotected sex Those requiring hemodialysis Infants born to HBV+ mothers Those with multiple tattoos and body piercings Health care workers Recipients of blood and blood products before 1984	Same as for HBV, especially IV drug users Recipients of blood and blood products before 1990 Recipients of organ transplants Recipients of artificial insemination

Copyright © 2027 by Elsevier, Inc. All rights are reserved, including those for text and data mining, AI training, and similar technologies.

	Hepatitis A	Hepatitis B	Hepatitis C
Age	All ages	More prevalent after puberty	More prevalent after puberty
Incubation period	2–6 weeks	1–6 months (average 60–90 days)	2 weeks to 6 months (average 6–9 weeks)
Duration of signs and symptoms	2 months	4–12 weeks	2–12 weeks
Carrier state	None	Yes	Yes
Complications	Rare	Chronicity Hepatocellular carcinoma Cirrhosis and liver failure Fulminant hepatitis	Chronicity: more than 50% Hepatocellular cancer Cirrhosis and liver failure
Serological markers	Anti-HAV IgM: indicative of acute infection Anti-HAV IgG: indicative of past exposure	HBsAg (surface antigen): indicator of infection Anti-HBs: recovery and noninfectivity; effective protection HBeAg (core antigen): marker of active infection Anti-HBe: signals onset of resolution Anti-HBc (core antigen): marker of recent infection: NOT protective HBV DNA: indicator of infection	Anti-HCV: indicator of infection; NOT protective HCV RNA: indicator of infection
Medications	None	Chronic cases with abnormal liver function tests: Interferon alpha-2b Lamivudine	With elevated ALT: Interferon alpha-2b Ribavirin
Immunoglobulin vaccine	Yes	Yes	No

29. from virus or bacterially contaminated stool or food or fomites to hands to mouth and fomites (inanimate objects) by poor hygiene and unsanitary toilet practices (e.g., not washing hands after bowel movement); examples include:
    - virus that has been excreted in stool of infected individual is ingested (as contaminated food or water) by another person
    - children with poor toileting behavior, particularly in large day care centers
    - poor handwashing in nursing homes
    - eating shellfish from contaminated water
30. It is an incomplete RNA virus that requires the presence of HBV so as to replicate.
31. (Table 17.5) by serological markers
32. (Table 17.5) by fecal-oral route
33. General signs and symptoms include:
    - preicteric stage: fatigue and malaise, anorexia and nausea, and general muscle aching; elevated serum levels of liver enzymes (AST, ALT)
    - icteric stage: jaundice; light-colored stool; dark urine and pruritic skin; tender, enlarged liver, causing mild aching pain; blood clotting times elevated in severe cases
    - posticteric stage: reduction in signs, may last for several weeks; depending on specific viral etiology
34. Hepatitis B has a relatively long incubation period, averaging about 2 months. Long incubation periods make it more difficult to track sources and contacts for infections. A carrier state is also common for HBV, in which the individual is asymptomatic but is contagious for the disease.
35. progressive destruction of liver tissue, leading eventually to liver failure
36. Causes include:
    - alcoholic liver disease
    - biliary cirrhosis: associated with immune disorders and disorders causing biliary obstruction such as stones or cystic fibrosis
    - postnecrotic cirrhosis: linked with chronic hepatitis or long-term exposure to toxic chemicals
    - metabolic: usually caused by storage disorders, such as hemochromatosis

Copyright © 2027 by Elsevier, Inc. All rights are reserved, including those for text and data mining, AI training, and similar technologies.

37. (Fig. 17.24) Liver demonstrates extensive diffuse fibrosis and loss of lobular organization. Nodules of regenerated hepatocytes may be present but are nonfunctional because the vascular network and biliary ducts are distorted. Fibrosis interferes with the blood supply. Bile may back up, causing ongoing inflammation and damage. Initial hepatomegaly is replaced by small, shrunken, and scarred liver.
38. Lost or impaired liver functions include:
    - decreased removal and conjugation of bilirubin
    - decreased bile production
    - impaired digestion and absorption of nutrients, especially fats and fat-soluble vitamins
    - decreased production of blood-clotting factors and plasma proteins
    - impaired glucose/glycogen metabolism
    - inadequate storage of iron and vitamin B_{12}
    - decreased inactivation of hormones, such as aldosterone and estrogen
    - decreased removal of toxic substances from the blood
39. (Table 17.6) Signs and symptoms include fatigue, anorexia; ascites; general edema; esophageal varices, hemorrhoids; splenomegaly; anemia; leukopenia, thrombocytopenia; increased bleeding, purpura; hepatic encephalopathy, tremors, confusion, coma; gynecomastia, impotence, irregular menses; jaundice; and pruritus.
40. (Fig. 17.27) blockage of blood flow through the liver leading to high pressure in the portal veins
41. (Figs. 17.27 and 17.28)
    - ascites, splenomegaly, esophageal varices
    - impaired respiration
    - increased risk of peritonitis
    - impaired digestion and absorption
42. Interventions include supportive or symptomatic treatments, such as avoiding fatigue and exposure to infection; dietary restrictions on protein and sodium; high carbohydrate intake and vitamin supplementation; use of diuretics to balance serum electrolytes; paracentesis to remove excess fluid; albumin transfusions; antimicrobials such as neomycin to remove intestinal flora; surgery for esophageal varices; and liver transplantation.

PANCREATITIS

43. gallstones and alcohol abuse
44. (Fig. 17.31) Pancreatitis results in premature activation of pancreatic enzymes inside the pancreatic duct, followed by autodigestion of pancreatic tissue. There is tissue necrosis and severe inflammation of pancreas. Leakage of enzymes into general circulation may cause shock, disseminated intravascular coagulation, and acute respiratory distress syndrome. Leakage of enzymes into the peritoneal cavity continues to destroy tissue and cause massive inflammation, leading to severe pain, hemorrhage and shock, peritonitis, and hypovolemic shock.
45. Signs and symptoms include severe epigastric or abdominal pain radiating to the back, which increases when supine; signs of shock, including low blood pressure, pallor, and sweating; rapid but weak pulse, low-grade fever; and abdominal distention and decreased bowel sounds.
46. Treatment includes stopping all oral intake; relieving bowel distention; treating shock and electrolyte imbalances; and prescribing analgesics but NOT morphine.

INTESTINAL DISORDERS

47. malabsorption syndrome, primarily in childhood; genetic factors resulting in defect in intestinal enzymes needed to complete digestion of gliadin, a breakdown product of gluten.
48. (Fig. 17.32*B*) The combination of a digestive block with an immunological response results in a toxic effect on the intestinal villi; villi atrophy, resulting in decreased enzyme production and reduced surface area for absorption of nutrients, resulting in malabsorption and malnutrition.
49. steatorrhea, muscle wasting, and failure to gain weight; irritability and malaise are common
50. Treatment is adopting a gluten-free diet, avoiding grains such as wheat, barley, and oats.
51. Crohn disease and ulcerative colitis are chronic inflammatory bowel diseases of unknown etiology that involve the inflammation and subsequent destruction of intestinal tissue.
52. (Table 17.7, Fig. 17.33).

	Crohn Disease	**Ulcerative Colitis**
Individuals at high risk	European ancestry, Ashkenazi Jews	European ancestry, Ashkenazi Jews, young adults (20s and 30s)
Etiology	Genetic basis; high familial tendency	Genetic basis; high familial tendency
Location of lesions	Terminal ileum; sometimes colon	Colon, rectum
Characteristics of lesions	Transmural: all layers "Skip" lesions Granuloma	Mucosa only: continuous Ulcerations

Copyright © 2027 by Elsevier, Inc. All rights are reserved, including those for text and data mining, AI training, and similar technologies.

	Crohn Disease	Ulcerative Colitis
Complications	Malabsorption; malnutrition Steatorrhea Adhesions; strictures Intestinal obstruction Fistulas and fissures	Malabsorption (rarely) Toxic megacolon leading to obstruction Iron deficient anemia
Signs and symptoms	Loose or semiformed stool Melena Cramping, abdominal pain Anorexia, weight loss, fatigue Delayed growth in children	Frequent watery stools with blood and mucus Cramping pain Fever Weight loss

53. Treatment includes identification and removal of stressors, antiinflammatory medications, antimotility agents, nutritional supplements, antimicrobials, immunotherapeutic agents, and surgical resection (ileostomy or colostomy).
54. (Fig. 17.35)
    - The appendiceal lumen becomes obstructed by a fecalith, gallstone, or foreign material or from twisting or spasm.
    - Fluid builds up inside the appendix and pathogens proliferate.
    - Inflammation with purulent exudate occurs, and appendix swells, compressing blood vessels.
    - Increasing pressure and congestion lead to ischemia and necrosis, resulting in increased permeability of the wall.
    - Bacteria and toxins escape through the wall into the area, resulting in abscess formation or localized bacterial peritonitis.
    - Abscess develops when adjacent omentum adheres to appendiceal surface in an attempt to wall off the inflammation.
    - Localized infection or peritonitis develops and may spread along peritoneal membranes.
    - Necrosis and gangrene develop in the appendiceal wall.
    - The appendix ruptures or perforates, releasing contents into the peritoneal cavity.
55.
    - general periumbilical pain
    - nausea and vomiting
    - increasing severity of pain, which becomes localized in lower right quadrant (LRQ)
    - LRQ tenderness
    - pain may subside temporarily following rupture
    - pain recurs with steady, severe abdominal pain
    - low-grade fever and leukocytosis
    - onset of peritonitis includes rigid abdomen, tachycardia, and hypotension
56. Complete Blood Count (CBC), ultrasound, CT scan, MRI
57. A diverticulum is a herniation or outpouching of the mucosa through the muscular layer of the colon. Diverticulitis refers to inflammation of the diverticula.
58. (Fig. 17.39) Warning signs vary depending on location of the tumor within the bowel.
    - ascending colon: liquid stool; occult blood or melena; anemia, fatigue; late palpable mass
    - transverse colon: semisolid stool; anemia, occult blood, change in bowel habits
    - descending colon: solid stool; constipation, discomfort; abdominal fullness and distention; red or dark blood in stool
    - rectum: solid stool; abdominal discomfort and cramps; ribbon or pellet stool; incomplete emptying; red blood on surface of stool
59. CBC, ultrasound, CT scan, MRI, colonoscopy and biopsy, x-ray and Positron Emission Tomography (PET)
60. (Fig. 17.41)
    A. Inguinal hernia, B. Volvulus, C. Intussusception, D. Tumor, E. Diverticulitis
61. (Fig. 17.42) Intestinal obstruction is a mechanical obstruction of the flow of the intestinal contents. Gases and fluids accumulate in the proximal area, distending the intestine. Increasingly strong contractions occur. Increasing intraluminal pressure leads to more secretions and compression of the veins, preventing absorption. Intestinal distention leads to persistent vomiting and loss of fluid and electrolytes, resulting in hypovolemia. If the obstruction is not removed, ischemia and necrosis of the intestinal wall may result, leading to potential gangrene, depending on the cause. There is decreased innervation and cessation of peristalsis (decrease in bowel sounds). There is rapid overgrowth of intestinal bacteria and production of endotoxins, which leak into peritoneal cavity (peritonitis) and the bloodstream (septicemia and bacteremia). In time, there is perforation and generalized peritonitis. If the obstruction is functional rather than mechanical, then peristalsis ceases, and there is distention of intestine. There are no reflex spasms. The rest of sequence is the same as above.
62. Signs and symptoms include:
    - mechanical obstruction of small intestine
    - severe, colicky abdominal pain
    - borborygmi (audible rumbling sounds) and intestinal rushes
    - vomiting and abdominal distention occur quickly

Copyright © 2027 by Elsevier, Inc. All rights are reserved, including those for text and data mining, AI training, and similar technologies.

- restlessness and sweating with tachycardia
- signs of dehydration, weakness, confusion, and shock
- in paralytic ileus, bowel sounds decrease or are absent and pain is steady
- large intestine obstruction: develops slowly and signs are mild
- constipation and mild lower abdominal pain
- abdominal distention, anorexia
- vomiting and more severe pain

63. inflammation of the peritoneal membranes
64. chemical irritation; bacterial invasion
65. (Fig. 17.44)
    - local inflammation of the peritoneum and omentum producing a thick, sticky exudate; abscess formation; reduction in peristalsis (attempts to keep inflammation, infection localized)
    - rapid dissemination of irritants or bacteria throughout abdomen with distention and reflex abdominal spasm (involvement of parietal peritoneum)
    - vasodilation and increased capillary permeability of peritoneal membrane; edema; leakage of fluid into peritoneal cavity ("third spacing"); hypovolemic shock
    - fluid becomes sequestered in peritoneal cavity; leaked fluid becomes purulent as infection spreads; nausea and vomiting from intestinal irritation and pain, adding to fluid/electrolyte loss
    - complications if intervention delayed; nerve conduction is impaired, peristalsis decreases leading to obstruction; movement of bacteria and toxins into bloodstream resulting in bacteremia and septicemia
66. Signs and symptoms include sudden and severe generalized abdominal pain, localized tenderness, pain increasing with movement (individual often restricts breathing), vomiting, signs of dehydration and hypovolemia, fever and leukocytosis, abdominal distention, rigid abdomen (involvement of parietal peritoneum), and decreased bowel sound (paralytic ileus and secondary obstruction).
67. Methods of diagnosis include: body fluid and urine analysis, CT scan, ultrasound and physical examination to evaluate tissue/organ damage.
68. Treatments include surgery and drainage of infection site, antimicrobial drugs, replacement therapy, and nasogastric suction to relieve distention.

CONSOLIDATION

69. (Table 17.3)
    i. antiinflammatory (e.g., inflammatory bowel disease [Crohn, ulcerative colitis])
    ii. antiemetic (e.g., acute gastritis, gastroenteritis)
    iii. antibolic (e.g., peptic ulcers, inflammatory bowel disease [Crohn, ulcerative colitis], diverticular disease, peritonitis)
    iv. acid reduction—proton pump inhibitor (e.g., hiatus hernia, gastroesophageal reflux disease, chronic gastritis)
    v. antidiarrheal e.g., gastroenteritis, dumping syndrome, inflammatory bowel disease [Crohn, ulcerative colitis])
    vi. laxative (e.g., diverticular disease)
    vii. coating agent (e.g., chronic gastritis, gastroesophageal reflux disease, peptic ulcer)

CHAPTER 18: Urinary System Disorders

1. See Fig. 18.1 of the text.
   A. Ribs, B. Adrenal gland, C. Renal artery, D. Kidney (left), E. Aorta, F. Ureter, G. Rectum, H. Ureteral opening, I. Trigone, J. Urethra, K. Penis, L. Prostate gland, M. Urinary bladder, N. Pelvis, O. Inferior vena cava, P. Hilum, Q. Renal vein
2. See Fig. 18.3*C* of the text.
   A. Afferent arteriole, B. Glomerular capillaries, C. Efferent arteriole, D. Distal convoluted tubules, E. Collecting duct, F. Arcuate vein, G. Urine flow, H. Peritubular capillaries, I. Loop of Henle, J. Arcuate artery, K. Proximal convoluted tubule
3. *cloudy:* may indicate the presence of large amounts of protein, blood cells, or bacteria and pus; *dark color:* may indicate hematuria, excessive bilirubin, or concentrated urine; *unpleasant or unusual odor:* may indicate infection or may result from certain dietary components or medications
4. (Fig. 18.6) blood (hematuria); protein (proteinuria, albuminuria); bacteria (bacteriuria); pus (pyuria); urinary casts; glucose and ketones
5. (Table 18.2) Diuretics are used to remove excess sodium ions and water from the body. They increase the excretion of water, which reduces fluid volume in tissues and blood. Examples: hydrochlorothiazide, furosemide.
6. (Fig. 18.7) Hemodialysis is provided in a hospital or dialysis center. A patient's blood moves via an implanted shunt through a dialysis machine, where exchange of wastes, fluid, and electrolytes takes place across a semipermeable membrane via ultrafiltration, diffusion, and osmosis and then is returned to the patient's bloodstream. Peritoneal dialysis is administered at home or in a dialysis unit and can be administered while the patient is asleep or ambulatory. Dialyzing fluid is instilled via catheter into the peritoneal cavity and allowed to remain there, facilitating exchanges of wastes and electrolytes by diffusion and osmosis across a semipermeable membrane; then the dialysate is drained from the cavity via gravity into a container.
7. Complications include an infected shunt or formation of blood clots, sclerosis and damage to blood vessels involved in the shunt, and increased risk of infection by hepatitis virus or human immunodeficiency virus (HIV)
8. Although rare, there is always the possibility that the equipment was not sterilized properly, and the dialysis patient will be exposed to these viruses.
9. Any invasive procedure such as dental scaling or extractions may introduce bacteria into the blood, resulting in a temporary bacteremia.
10. (Fig. 18.8) Predisposing factors include prostatic hypertrophy and urinary retention in older men,

Copyright © 2027 by Elsevier, Inc. All rights are reserved, including those for text and data mining, AI training, and similar technologies.

congenital abnormalities in children, incomplete bladder emptying, reduced fluid intake, impaired blood supply to the bladder, and immobility. Women are anatomically more vulnerable to infection because of the shortness and width of the urethra, the proximity of the urethra to the anus, and the frequent irritation to the tissues caused by sexual activity, tampons, bubble bath, and deodorants.

11. Manifestations of cystitis include lower abdominal pain; dysuria, urgency, frequency, and nocturia; systemic signs of infection (fever, malaise, nausea, and leukocytosis); cloudy urine with an unusual odor; and urinalysis indicating bacteruria. Manifestations of pyelonephritis include signs and symptoms of cystitis, pain associated with renal disease (dull aching pain in lower back), more marked systemic signs, and urinalysis similar to that of cystitis plus the addition of urinary casts.
12. (Figs. 18.9 and 18.10) Antistreptococcal antibodies, resulting from earlier infection, create an antigen-antibody complex that lodges in the glomerular capillaries, activating the complement to cause an inflammatory response in both kidneys. This leads to increased capillary permeability and cell proliferation, resulting in leakage of protein and RBCs into the glomerular filtrate. When inflammation is severe, it interferes with filtration, causing decreased glomerular filtration rate (GFR) and fluid retention. Acute renal failure is possible if blood flow is sufficiently impaired. Renin secretion is likely to be triggered, leading to elevated blood pressure and edema. If the process becomes chronic, the kidneys will be scarred.
13. Signs and symptoms include:
    - dark and cloudy urine
    - facial and periorbital edema, followed by generalized edema
    - elevated blood pressure
    - flank pain
    - general signs of inflammation, including malaise, fatigue, headache, anorexia, and nausea
    - oliguria
14.
    - blood tests showing elevated serum urea and creatinine, elevated antistreptococcal antibodies (ASO and ASK), and decreased complement level
    - metabolic acidosis with low serum pH and bicarbonate
    - proteinuria, gross hematuria, and erythrocyte casts
15. sodium restriction, decreased protein and fluid intake; drug treatment includes glucocorticoids to reduce inflammation; antihypertensives to reduce blood pressure
16.
    - abnormality in the glomerular capillaries and increased permeability resulting in proteinuria (albuminuria)
    - hypoalbuminemia leading to generalized edema due to decreased plasma osmotic pressure
    - low or normal blood pressure with hypovolemia or elevated depending on angiotensin levels
    - hypovolemia leading to aldosterone secretion and more severe edema
    - high levels of blood cholesterol and lipoprotein in the urine due to unknown factors, possibly liver response to protein loss in the urine
17. *most significant sign:* massive edema or anasarca; *potential consequences include:*
    - weight gain
    - pallor
    - anorexia
    - dyspnea
    - decreased exercise tolerance
    - skin breakdown and subsequent infection
18. glucocorticoids, angiotensin-converting enzyme (ACE) inhibitors, and antihypertensives
19. Causative factors include excessive amounts of insoluble salts in the filtrate (e.g., hypercalcemia due to hyperparathyroidism, hyperuricemia due to gout or cancer chemotherapy).
20. Small stones that are "passed" will be visible and can be analyzed for content.
21. Signs and symptoms include flank pain due to distention of the renal capsule, renal colic (intense spasms of pain in the flank area radiating into the groin), perhaps accompanied by nausea and vomiting, cool moist skin, and rapid pulse; confirmed by radiological examination.
22. buildup of urine due to obstruction of outflow, causing a dilated area proximal to the obstruction in either ureter or kidney and resulting in tissue atrophy and necrosis
23. (Fig. 18.12B) secondary complication of calculi, tumors, scar tissue in the kidney or ureter, stenosis or kinking of the ureter, and untreated prostatic enlargement; developmental defects
24. smoking
25. "arteriosclerosis" of renal vasculature
26. (Fig. 18.14) primary vascular changes in the kidney or secondary to essential hypertension, diabetes mellitus (see diabetic nephropathy and Fig. 25.6 in Chapter 25), or another condition
27.
    - Vesicoureteral reflux: due to a defective valve in the bladder
    - Agenesis: failure of one kidney to develop
    - Hypoplasia: failure of kidney to develop to normal size
    - Ectopic kidney: kidney and ureters are displaced out of normal position
    - Fusion of two kidneys during development: "horseshoe" kidney

RENAL FAILURE

28. (Fig. 18.16, Table 18.3) Causes include bilateral kidney disease, such as glomerulonephritis; severe and prolonged circulatory shock or heart failure; sepsis; nephrotoxins; ischemia; pyelonephritis; and occasionally mechanical obstructions such as calculi,

Copyright © 2027 by Elsevier, Inc. All rights reserved, including those for text and data mining, AI training, and similar technologies.

blood clots, or tumors, only when affecting both kidneys (bilateral).

29. Reverse the primary problem quickly and provide dialysis.
30. (Table 18.3) Causes include nephrosclerosis, diabetes mellitus, nephrotoxins, chronic exposure, chronic bilateral kidney inflammation or infection, and polycystic disease.
31. (Fig. 18.17) Renal insufficiency is the second stage of chronic renal failure when about 75% of the nephrons are lost. End-stage renal failure or uremia occurs when more than 90% of nephrons are lost and GFR is negligible.
32. (Table 18.3, Fig. 18.16)
    i. fluid, wastes retained; all body systems affected; oliguria or anuria; hypocalcemia, hyperphosphatemia, hyponatremia, hyperkalemia; acidosis
    ii. congestive heart failure (CHF), arrhythmias, hypertension
    iii. encephalopathy (lethargy, memory lapses, seizures, tremors)
    iv. osteodystrophy (Fig. 18.18), osteoporosis, and tetany
    v. impotence and decreased libido in men; menstrual irregularities in women
    vi. dry, pruritic, and hyperpigmented skin; easy bruising; uremic frost in terminal stage
33.
    i. GFR declines and tubule function is lost
    ii. potassium retained as GFR decreases
    iii. decreased renal activation of vitamin D leading to decreased GI calcium absorption; high phosphate levels
    iv. decreased GFR
    v. decreased production of erythropoietin leading to decreased RBC production; bone marrow depression
    vi. red bone marrow function depressed by altered blood chemistry that leads to decreased platelet production
    vii. increased blood volume due to decreased GFR
    viii. increased blood volume; increased renin secretion
    ix. electrolyte imbalances, particularly hypocalcemia and hyperkalemia
    x. increased blood volume and increased blood pressure
    xi. due to development of heart failure
    xii. due to accumulation of nitrogenous wastes in blood, particularly urea: acidosis
    xiii. due to hypocalcemia and encephalopathy
    xiv. due to bone demineralization (hypocalcemia stimulates secretion of parathyroid hormone [PTH], which causes bone resorption)
    xv. abnormal metabolism of hormones; increased wastes in serum
    xvi. due to presence of uremic frost
    xvii. urea catabolism; ammonia being excreted in respirations
    xviii. due to hypocalcemia, resulting in increased secretion of PTH
34. Most drugs are excreted primarily via the kidney. With renal failure, the rate of drug excretion decreases, resulting in accumulation of the medication. This can result in increased adverse, potentially toxic drug effects.
35. answer to crossword puzzle

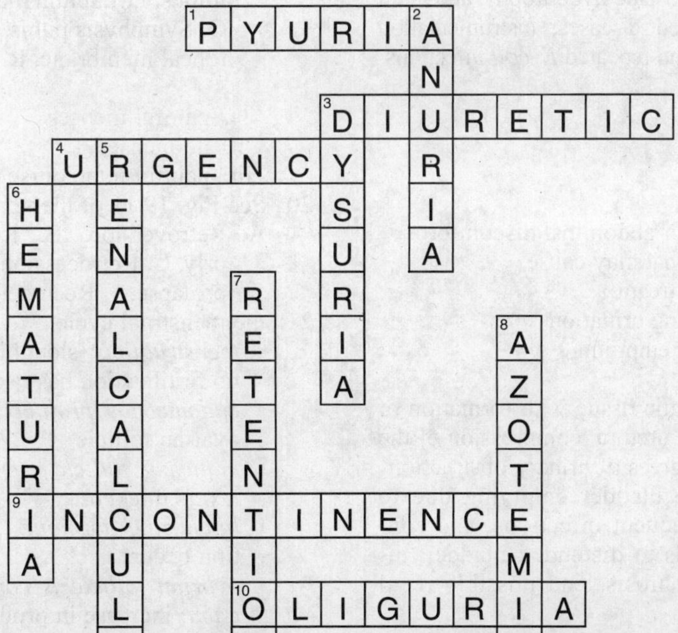

Copyright © 2027 by Elsevier, Inc. All rights are reserved, including those for text and data mining, AI training, and similar technologies.

CHAPTER 19: Reproductive System Disorders

1.
- *males:* changes in sperm or semen, hormonal abnormalities, physical obstruction of the sperm passage
- *females:* hormonal imbalances resulting from altered function of hypothalamus, anterior pituitary, or ovaries; structural abnormalities; obstruction of fallopian tubes; abnormal vaginal pH; cigarette smoking

MALE

2. See Fig. 19.1 of the text.
   A. Parietal peritoneal membrane, B. Ureter, C. Surface of urinary bladder, D. Seminal vesicle, E. Urinary bladder opened, F. Ampulla, G. Ejaculatory duct, H. Prostatic urethra, I. Prostate gland, J. Rectum, K. Membranous urethra, L. Bulbourethral gland, M. Spongy urethra, N. Penis, O. Ductus deferens, P. Urethra, Q. Epididymis, R. Testis, S. Seminiferous tubules, T. Scrotum, U. Prepuce, V. Glans penis
3.
   i. urethral opening on the ventral surface of the penis
   ii. urethral opening on the dorsal surface of the penis
   iii. undescended testes (Fig. 19.2)
   iv. excessive fluid collects between the layers of the tunica vaginalis (Fig. 19.3A)
   v. cyst containing fluid and sperm that develops between the testes and the epididymis
   vi. dilated vein in the spermatic cord (Fig. 19.3B)
   vii. development of fibrous scar tissue on the penis which causes a significant bend and/or pain
4. young men in association with urinary tract infections, older men with benign prostatic hypertrophy, and in all men: sexually transmitted diseases, instrumentation such as catheterization, and repeated *E. coli* infections
5. *Escherichia coli*
6.
   - dysuria
   - urinary frequency
   - urgency
   - low back pain or lower abdominal discomfort
   - severe inflammation that may cause:
     - decreased urinary stream
     - hesitancy in initiating urination
     - incomplete bladder emptying
     - nocturia
7. hyperplasia of the prostatic tissue with formation of nodules surrounding the urethra, compression of the urethra, and variable degrees of urinary obstruction
8. (Fig. 19.5) Incomplete bladder emptying due to obstruction leads to frequent infections, and continued obstruction leads to distended bladder, dilated ureters, hydronephrosis, and possible renal damage.
9. hesitancy, dribbling, decreased force of the urinary stream, frequency, nocturia, recurrent infections
10. A single cause has not been determined. Genetic mutations, high androgen and insulin-like growth factors, and recurrent prostatic infections appear to be causative factors. It is common in men of North American and northern European descent. There is a higher incidence in the black population.
11. Warning signs include hard nodule in the periphery of the gland on rectal examination, elevated prostate specific antigen (not diagnostic, also occurs with benign prostatic hypertrophy), and signs of urinary obstruction.
12. metastasis to bone
13. Serum tests for prostate specific antigen (PSA) and prostatic acid phosphatase, ultrasound, MRI, CT scan, PET scan, and biopsy.
14. Use of antitestosterone drugs that act as testosterone blocking agents may be suggested to reduce hormonal effects on androgen-sensitive tumors.
15. Risk factors include familial incidence, cryptorchidism, infection, and trauma.
16. Manifestations include hard, painless, usually unilateral mass; enlarged or "heavy" testes; dull aching pain in the lower abdomen; hydrocele or epididymitis and gynecomastia.
17. Treatment includes a combination of surgery, radiation, and chemotherapy. High dose chemotherapy can also be used along with a stem cell transplant to replace cells destroyed by high chemical dosing.

FEMALE

18. See Fig. 19.8A of the text.
    A. Ovary, B. Fallopian tube, C. Fimbriae, D. Coccyx, E. Posterior fornix, F. Cervix, G. Vagina, H. Rectum, I. Anus, J. Vaginal orifice, K. Labium minus, L. Labium majus, M. Clitoris, N. Urethra, O. Symphysis pubis, P. Urinary bladder, O. Peritoneal membrane, R. Uterus
19.
    i. painful menses
    ii. no menses
    iii. painful intercourse
20. See Fig. 19.11 of the text.
    A. Retroversion, B. Retroflexion-flexion posteriorly, C. Retrocession, D. Anteflexion, E. Uterine prolapse, F. Rectocele, G. Cystocele
21. the menstrual cycle:
    - *menstruation:* sloughing of endometrial tissue if no fertilization has taken place
    - *endometrial proliferation stage:* maturation of ovarian follicle
    - *maturing follicle secretes estrogen:* endometrial layers thicken
    - *luteinizing hormone (LH) levels increase:* ovulation occurs
    - *ovarian follicle is converted into the corpus luteum:* increase in production of progesterone
    - *progesterone increases development of endometrial blood vessels* in preparation of fertilized ovum

Copyright © 2027 by Elsevier, Inc. All rights are reserved, including those for text and data mining, AI training, and similar technologies.

If fertilization of the egg does not occur, hormone levels drop, and the corpus luteum and endometrium begin to degenerate, eventually sloughing off and beginning the cycle again.

Endometriosis

22. (Fig. 19.12) the presence of endometrial tissue outside of the uterus on structures such as the ovaries, ligaments, or colon
23. (Fig. 19.12) The ectopic endometrium responds to cyclic hormonal changes just as the normal uterus does; there is no exit point for shed tissue and blood, which causes local inflammation and pain, recurring with each menstrual cycle. Fibrous tissue may cause adhesions and obstruction of involved structures, such as urinary bladder, colon, and ovary (infertility).
24. dysmenorrhea
25. Treatment involves hormonal suppression of endometrial tissue and surgical removal of ectopic tissue.

Vaginal Candidiasis

26. Predisposing factors include antimicrobial therapy for an unrelated bacterial infection, immunodeficiency states, and increased glycogen or glucose in secretions (e.g., from use of oral contraceptives and diabetes mellitus).
27.
    - red and swollen pruritic mucous membranes
    - thick, white, curdlike discharge
    - white patches adhering to the vaginal wall
    - dysuria
    - dyspareunia

Pelvic Inflammatory Disease (PID)

28. an infection of the reproductive tract, particularly the fallopian tubes and ovaries; includes cervicitis, endometritis, salpingitis, and oophoritis
29. Predisposing factors for PID include sexually transmitted disease, prior episode of vaginitis or cervicitis, insertion of an IUD or other instrument, septicemia, or peritoneal infections.
30. (Fig. 19.13)
    - vaginitis or cervicitis of polymicrobial etiology
    - ascending inflammation and infection from uterus into fallopian tubes, causing edema and obstruction
    - exudate contaminates ovary and surrounding tissue
    - peritonitis may develop, with pelvic abscess formation
    - potential septicemia
    - adhesions and strictures common sequelae, leading to infertility or ectopic pregnancy, as well as affecting surrounding structures such as the colon
31. Manifestations of PID include:
    - lower abdominal pain, which may be sudden and severe or gradually increasing in intensity
    - steady pain that increases with walking
    - tenderness
    - purulent discharge
    - dysuria
    - fever and leukocytosis
    - abdominal distention and rigidity indicate peritonitis
32. Complications if untreated include pelvic abscess, septicemia, death, adhesions, and strictures of surrounding tissues: infertility or ectopic pregnancy.
33. aggressive antimicrobial therapy

BREAST CANCER

34. Risk factors include being older than 50, having a genetic predisposition, familial occurrence, hormonal influences (especially exposure to high estrogen levels), long menstrual cycles, and delay or absence of a first pregnancy. Exogenous estrogen in oral contraceptives or postmenopausal supplements as a cause is controversial. Other factors include fibrocystic disease, prior carcinoma in the uterus or other breast, and radiation of the chest.
35.
    - majority arise from malignant transformation of breast tissue
    - local infiltration of surrounding tissues and adherence to skin causing dimpling
    - spread to nearby axillary lymph nodes early
    - widespread dissemination follows quickly, including metastases to lung, brain, bone, and liver
36. Manifestations include:
    - single small, hard, painless nodule in the breast; freely moveable in early stages
    - dimpling of the skin, fixation of the nodule to the skin, retraction of or discharge from the nipples, and change in breast contour
37. Therapeutic interventions include surgical removal of the tumor with minimal tissue loss or a more radical mastectomy combined with radiation, chemotherapy and hormone therapy and immunotherapy using monoclonal antibodies. Surgical removal of some lymph nodes is usually warranted. The ovaries are removed if the tumor is responsive to hormones. New classes of targeted drugs are also being developed and used in therapies primarily focusing on the suppression of cancer cell growth factors.
38. Early detection measures include breast self-examination regularly for all women older than 20 years and mammography, especially if family history warrants and routinely after age 40.

CERVICAL CANCER

39. Increased use of Pap smear for screening has had two results:
    - Early detection allows for effective treatment at an early stage, improving prognosis and survival.
    - Early detection while cancer is still *in situ;* more cases are detected earlier in a younger population.
40. Individuals at high risk include Hispanic American women, those with multiple sexual partners, those with promiscuous partners, early sexual intercourse in teen years, a history of STDs, and environmental factors

Copyright © 2027 by Elsevier, Inc. All rights are reserved,
including those for text and data mining, AI training, and similar technologies.

such as smoking cigarettes, long time use of oral contraceptives, immunosuppression and family history.

41. (Fig. 19.18)
    - cervical dysplasia—mild
    - cervical dysplasia—severe
    - malignant neoplasm
    - carcinoma *in situ*
    - invasive carcinoma
42. asymptomatic early but detectable by Pap smear; slight bleeding or watery discharge; anemia or weight loss
43. Biopsy confirms the diagnosis. Surgery and radiation constitute the usual treatment measures with chemotherapy in the later stages. When chemotherapy is used, a combination of two drugs is sometimes used such as Gemcitabine and Cisplatin.

ENDOMETRIAL CANCER

44. Individuals at high risk include those with a history of increased estrogen levels, postmenopausal women who have taken exogenous estrogen, infertile women, those who took sequential oral contraceptives early, obese women, those with diabetes, and those with hypertension.
45.
    - endometrial hyperplasia of the glandular epithelium (due to excessive estrogen stimulation)
    - slow growth and infiltration of uterine wall
    - continued growth results in tumor mass filling the interior of the uterus and infiltrating and extending through the wall into surrounding structures
    - grading and staging determined by degree of cell differentiation/undifferentiation (grade) and extent of spread (stage)
46. Manifestations include painless vaginal bleeding or spotting (early sign), palpable mass, discomfort or pressure in the lower abdomen, and bleeding following intercourse (late sign).
47. surgery and radiation therapy

SEXUALLY TRANSMITTED DISEASES (STDs)

48. See Table 19.1.

CHAPTER 20: Neoplasms and Cancer

1.
    i. a tumor, a cellular growth that is no longer responding to normal body controls
    ii. tumor of differentiated cells that reproduce at higher-than-normal rate but do not spread
    iii. tumor of undifferentiated, nonfunctional cells that reproduce rapidly, infiltrate surrounding areas, and may spread by metastases to other organs and tissues
    iv. malignant tumors of epithelial tissue
    v. malignant tumors of connective tissue
    vi. growth of undifferentiated cells of varying size and shape
2. normal organization, growth inhibition, cell-to-cell communications—all absent (alternate answers: cell membranes, surface antigens are altered)
3. (Table 20.1)

	Benign Tumor	Malignant Tumor
Pancreas	Adenoma	Adenocarcinoma
Fat	Lipoma	Liposarcoma
Bone	Osteoma	Osteosarcoma
Liver	Hepatoma	Hepatocarcinoma
Cartilage	Chondroma	Chondrosarcoma
Skin	Epithelioma	Carcinoma; melanoma

4. (Table 20.2)

	Benign Tumors	Malignant Tumors
Cells	Similar in appearance to normal cells Differentiated Mitosis normal	Varied in size and shape with large nuclei Many undifferentiated Mitosis increased and atypical nuclei present
Growth	Relatively slow Cells adhere in one mass No invasion of tissue Usually encapsulated	Rapid growth Cells lack adhesion, infiltrate adjacent tissue No capsule
Spread	Remain localized	Invade nearby tissues and may metastasize to distance sites through blood and lymph vessels
Systemic effects	Rare—except in CNS	Often present
General prognosis	Life-threatening in certain locations (e.g., brain)	Destroy local tissue function if untreated Many metastasize to vital organs, causing death if not treated

CNS, central nervous system

5. Regarding cellular aging, telomeres are protective caps found at the ends of chromosomes that naturally shorten with each cell division. The enzyme telomerase works to counteract this shortening by maintaining the length of telomeres. Scientists use the length of telomeres to estimate a cell's age and determine its remaining capacity for replication.

Copyright © 2027 by Elsevier, Inc. All rights are reserved, including those for text and data mining, AI training, and similar technologies.

6.
   i. ischemia, necrosis, and areas of inflammation around the tumor; potential for infection
   ii. blockage of secretion or normal flow of air (bronchi), food (GI tract), blood, or lymph depending on location
   iii. pain and loss of function
   iv. hemorrhage, inflammation, necrosis
   v. loss of normal tissue function
7.
   i. anorexia, fatigue, pain, stress, nutrient trapping, altered metabolism, and cachectic factors produced by macrophages
   ii. anorexia, decreased appetite and food intake, chronic bleeding, and bone marrow depression
   iii. host resistance decline; tissue breakdown and diminished immune system function; immobility
   iv. local invasion/erosion of blood vessels by tumor; bone marrow depression, and hypoproteinemia
8. additional problems associated with certain tumors (e.g., bronchogenic carcinoma cells producing ACTH, causing manifestations of Cushing syndrome)
9.
   i. indicator of effects of chemotherapy and radiation; hemoglobin and erythrocyte counts may be low—often a general sign of cancer
   ii. tests of blood and bodily fluids for tissue enzymes or hormones associated with particular cancers (e.g., carcinoembryonic antigen, human chorionic gonadotropin, prostate-specific antigen tests)
   iii. signs of abnormal growth or changes in organs and tissues
   iv. histopathological confirmation of diagnosis of malignancy
10. Malignant tumor cells lack cohesiveness and easily separate from the growing tumor mass; if invasive and eroding blood or lymphatic vessels, tumor cells can enter the circulation and reach distant sites. This is called *metastasis.*
11. Grading reflects the degree of differentiation or undifferentiation (degree of malignancy) of the tumor cells. Staging is the classification of tumors that reflects the extent of disease, *i.e.,* size of primary tumor, extent of lymph node spread, and metastasis (as in breast cancer).
12. (Fig. 20.8) Initiating factors cause the first irreversible cellular changes in the process of carcinogenesis. Promoters cause additional changes in DNA, resulting in less differentiation and greater rate of mitosis.
13. (Table 20.3)
   i. viruses: hepatitis virus (hepatic cancer)
   ii. radiation: (skin cancer)
   iii. chemical exposure: (lung cancer)
   iv. chronic irritation or inflammation: ulcerative colitis (breast cancer)
   v. increasing age: (many cancers are more common in older people)
   vi. diet: high-fat diet (colon cancer)
   vii. hormones: estrogen (endometrial cancer)
   viii. genetics: chromosomal abnormalities (leukemia)
14. (see also Chapter 7) Malignant tumors often have altered “nonself” antigens on their surface, which, if detected early, may invoke an immune response that prevents the growth and spread of the tumor. If the immune system is compromised or deficient (e.g., in people with AIDS), then transformed cells go undetected until sufficient growth has occurred to establish the tumor.
15. Radiation, surgery, and chemotherapy are often used in combination to completely eradicate local tumor and treat and/or prevent metastases. Biological modifiers and hormones may be used to limit the growth of specific tumors.
16. curative: used if tumor is small and localized; palliative: in advanced cancer, intended to reduce the manifestations and complications related to the cancer; prophylactic: used to prevent metastasis
17. Radiation causes mutations in the tumor cell DNA, preventing mitosis and tumor growth and causing immediate cell death; it also damages blood vessels, cutting off tumor blood supply.
18. Antimitotic agents, antimetabolites, alkylating agents, and some antibiotics interfere with protein synthesis and DNA replication at different points in the tumor cell cycle, therefore decreasing growth of the tumor.
19. Radiation and chemotherapy are most effective against reproducing cells, both normal and malignant because of their effects on DNA replication. Therefore normal cells that are dividing regularly are at the greatest risk (e.g., skin, GI tract mucosa, bone marrow, and gonads). Adverse effects include bone marrow depression (resulting in anemia, infections, bleeding, etc.), nausea and vomiting, and hair loss.
20. 1) Effects of the cancer itself: This includes issues like anorexia (loss of appetite), pain, or altered metabolism caused by the disease. 2) Effects of chemotherapy or radiation: Treatments can lead to side effects such as stomatitis (inflammation of the mouth), nausea, vomiting, or diarrhea, all of which can impair nutrient intake and absorption. 3) Psychological factors: Conditions like fear or anxiety can also contribute to malnutrition in these patients.
21. Biologic response modifiers are agents that augment the natural immune response to improve immune surveillance and removal of abnormal cells
22. Gene therapy treatment is designed to: replace mutated genes with healthy ones, inactivate mutated genes, introduce new genes.
23. sex hormones when the tumor growth is dependent on, or accelerated by, such hormones; hormone blocking agents, often effective in reducing tumors and preventing recurrences; angiogenesis inhibitor to prevent enhanced blood supply to tumors by preventing endothelial cell growth; analgesics for pain management; narcotics as pain intensity increases
24. basal cell carcinoma

Copyright © 2027 by Elsevier, Inc. All rights are reserved,
including those for text and data mining, AI training, and similar technologies.

25.

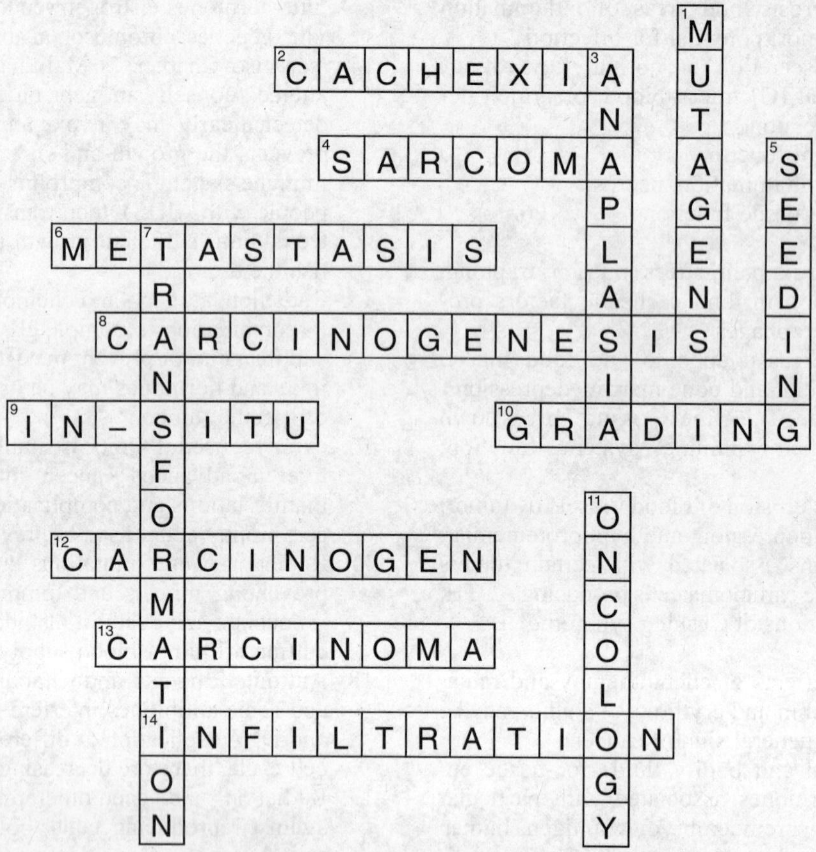

CHAPTER 21: Congenital and Genetic Disorders

1. Congenital defects refer to disorders present at birth; they include genetic (inherited) as well as developmental disorders.
2. errors in chromosomal duplication or reassembly during meiosis, resulting in abnormal placement of part of a chromosome (translocation), altered structure (deletion), or abnormal number of chromosomes
3. agents that cause damage during embryonic or fetal development; often difficult to define
4. Inherited disorders are any disorders resulting from abnormalities or damage to the genetic makeup, whereas chromosomal defects usually result from errors during meiosis when the chromosomes are segregating, when the DNA fragments are displaced or lost and therefore could involve many genes.
5. Autosomal recessive disorders: both parents must pass on the defective gene to produce an affected child. Autosomal dominant disorders: an affected parent has a 50% chance to pass the disorder to a child. X-linked dominant disorders: dominant allele carried on the X chromosome—males and females can be affected. X-linked recessive disorders: alleles carried by the X chromosome—manifested in heterozygous males—heterozygous females are carriers.
6. (Fig. 21.1)
   i. monosomy: when one member of a chromosome pair is lost during meiosis
   ii. trisomy: when there is extra duplication of one member of a chromosome pair, yielding three chromosomes instead of two
7. (Box 21.1) Multifactorial disorders occur when a combination of factors is responsible for the congenital disorder, *i.e.,* polygenic—caused by multiple genes or inherited tendency that is expressed following exposure to environmental factors. Examples include anencephaly, cleft lip and palate, clubfoot.
8. (Fig. 21.6) The most critical time for development is the first 2 months of gestation, when organogenesis occurs. Exposure to damaging substances may cause developmental abnormality, premature birth, high risk of further illness in the infant, and increased risk of sudden infant death syndrome. The effects of exposure depend on the stage of development at the precise time of the exposure.
9. Difficulties encountered during or after birth that may temporarily deprive the newborn of oxygen can cause brain damage (e.g., cerebral palsy).
10. maternal age over 35
11. A carrier of an infectious disease is contagious and can pass the infection to others. A carrier of a genetic disorder is heterozygous for that particular disorder and

Copyright © 2027 by Elsevier, Inc. All rights are reserved, including those for text and data mining, AI training, and similar technologies.

usually does not have any manifestations of the disorder; he may pass the faulty gene on to his children.

12. autosomal recessive and X-linked recessive disorders
13. heterozygous; does not usually become symptomatic
14. (Fig. 21.4)
    i. father
    ii. 50%
    iii. 0%—there is no carrier state in autosomal dominant disorders; an individual with the faulty gene has the disorder
15. (Fig. 21.4)
    i. both
    ii. 75%
16. (Fig. 21.4)
    i. a) neither b) mother c) both
    ii. a) 0% b) 50% c) 100% d) 50%
17. (Fig. 21.4)
    i. a) neither b) both c) both
    ii. a) 25% b) 50% c) 100% d) 50%
18. (Fig. 21.4)
    i. a) father b) mother c) mother
    ii. a) 50% b) 50% c) 50% d) 50%
19. (Fig. 21.4)
    i. homozygous
    ii. both
    iii. 25%
    iv. 50%
20. (Fig. 21.4)
    i. a) both b) neither c) neither
    ii. a) 100% b) 0% c) 0% d) 100%
21. (Fig. 21.4)
    Referring to Square A:
    i. a) neither b) mother
    ii. 25%
    iii. male
    iv. 25%—female
    v. a) 25% b) 25%
    Referring to Square B:
    i. a) father b) neither c) mother
    ii. a) 100% b) 0% c) 0% d) 0%
22. (Fig. 21.4) There is a 25% chance of a female with the disorder.
23. (Fig. 21.4)
    i. Xd Y
    ii. mother
    iii. daughter—0%; son—50%
    iv. brother—sex-linked disorder; for a female to be affected, father would have the disorder
    v. 50% of sisters will be carriers, 0% of brothers
24. (See Box 21.1)
25. (Fig. 21.1C) Down syndrome is a chromosomal disorder that is diagnosed prenatally through amniocentesis and karyotyping. The karyotype of an individual with Down syndrome is trisomy 21.
26. Down syndrome is trisomy 21, which results in numerous defects in physical and mental development, including hypotonic muscles, loose joints, cervical instability, delayed developmental states, cognitive impairment, and delayed sexual development. Miscellaneous other conditions may be present, including visual, hearing, and digestive problems; celiac disease; congenital heart disease; decreased resistance to infection; and a high risk of leukemia.
27. Individuals with Down syndrome may have a small head and flat facial profiles, slanted eyes, Brushfield's spots in the irises, a mouth that tends to hang open, a large protruding tongue and high arched palate, and small hands with single palmar crease. The muscles tend to be hypotonic, the joints are loose, cervical abnormalities and instability are often evident, and stature is short. Developmental stages are delayed, all children are cognitively impaired, but the severity of impairment varies with the individual, and early stimulation programs are helpful. Sexual development is often delayed or incomplete, many children have an assortment of other problems, including visual problems (cataracts, strabismus), hearing problems, obstructions in the digestive tract, celiac disease, congenital heart defects, decreased resistance to infection (immune deficit), and a high risk of developing leukemia.
28. *Turner Syndrome*—Also known as monosomy X, occurs when only one sex chromosome, the X chromosome, is present. This person has only 45 chromosomes, resulting in a variety of manifestations in females including: slow growth and no growth spurt at puberty, failure to begin sex changes at puberty, sex development stalls in teenage years, early end of menstrual cycle, inability to conceive naturally.
29. *Klinefelter Syndrome*—Also known as polysomy X, an extra X chromosome is present (XXY), resulting in a total of 47 chromosomes in each cell. Not all males show signs and are diagnosed but typically includes reduced muscular strength, tall stature, delayed puberty, broad hips and enlarged breasts, small testicles and low testosterone, weak bones, reduced sex drive, infertility, increased belly fat, and cognitive deficits.

CHAPTER 22: Complications of Pregnancy

1. embryonic stage: 3 to 8–10 weeks after fertilization; fetus: the term is used after 8 to 10 weeks; organogenesis: during embryonic stage, all organs are formed by the end of 8 weeks
2. low birth weight, increased irritability, increased risk of stillbirth, increased risk of placenta previa and abruption placentae
3. human chorionic gonadotropin; accurate only in first 10 weeks, then placenta takes over
4. a) milk production; iv. lactation b) pregnancy; i. gestation c) inflammation of uterine lining; v. endometritis d) number of pregnancies; ii. gravidity e) number of viable pregnancies; iii. parity
5.
    i. ectopic pregnancy: tubal pregnancy, when the fertilized ovum implants outside the uterus
    ii. preeclampsia and eclampsia: pregnancy-induced hypertension
    iii. gestational diabetes mellitus: increased glucose intolerance and increased blood glucose levels

Copyright © 2027 by Elsevier, Inc. All rights are reserved, including those for text and data mining, AI training, and similar technologies.

iv. placenta previa: when the placenta is implanted in the lower uterus or over the os cervical
v. abruptio placentae: premature separation of the placenta from the uterine wall
vi. thromboembolism and thrombophlebitis: clot formation in the veins of the legs or pelvis and potential for embolization if clot breaks free
vii. disseminated intravascular coagulation: increased activation of clotting mechanism, usually not a primary problem; however, can be a serious complication resulting in diffuse blood clots and consumption of clotting factors
viii. Rh incompatibility: can develop when Rh factor antigens on fetal red blood cells differ from those on maternal red blood cells; immune response of Rh-negative mother to Rh-positive fetal antigens, resulting in anti-Rh antibodies in the maternal bloodstream, *i.e.,* maternal anti-Rh sensitization with potential for hemolytic disease during subsequent pregnancies
ix. infections: puerperal infection (childbed fever); cervical lacerations or episiotomy repairs are vulnerable to infection; predisposition to endometritis—may spread to cause pelvic cellulitis or peritonitis
x. adolescent pregnancy: intrauterine growth retardation, maternal anemia, pregnancy-induced hypertension

6. (Fig. 22.2) Rh-negative mother exposed to Rh-positive blood via transfusion or pregnancy with Rh-positive fetus; immune response, anti-Rh sensitization resulting in potential for hemolytic disease in subsequent Rh-positive pregnancies
7. RhoGAM is Rh immunoglobulin, containing anti-Rh antibodies; when given to an Rh-negative woman who has not been previously sensitized, it confers temporary passive immunity and thus prevents maternal sensitization to Rh antigen.
8. Teenager has their own nutritional needs to be met, especially calcium, protein, and iron; teenager may not seek adequate prenatal care; lack of adequate nutrition for both teenager and fetus; woman's pelvis may be too small, increasing risk during labor and delivery; pregnancy-induced hypertension.

CHAPTER 23 Complications of Adolescence

1. Generally considered to begin with the development of secondary sex characteristics—age 10 to 12—and continues until physical growth is completed at about age 18.
2.

Height	Weight	BMI	N, Ov, Ob
4′7″	130	30.2	Ob
4′7″	100	23.2	N
4′11″	100	20.2	N
5′2″	140	25.6	Ob
5′7″	180	28.2	Ob
5′7″	210	32.9	Ob

BMI, Body mass index; *N,* normal; *Ob,* obese; *Ov,* overweight.

3. type 2 diabetes mellitus, elevated blood cholesterol/lipid levels, increased blood pressure
4. presence of significant abdominal fat mass resulting in an increased waistline measurement, changes in glucose and lipoprotein metabolism
5.
   a) condition characterized by alternating "binge and purge" behavior; iv. bulimia nervosa
   b) extreme weight loss due to self-starvation; iii. anorexia nervosa
   c) demineralization of bone; i. osteoporosis
   d) bone infection; ii. osteomyelitis
6. A. Lordosis, B. Kyphosis, C. Scoliosis
7. minor trauma such as a fracture or soft tissue injury; sickle cell anemia
8. The pathophysiology of osteomyelitis includes (1) accumulation of local purulent exudate, which destroys the bone in the damaged area, causing severe pain due to pressure on the nerves; if the fluid pressure is severe, may cause separation of the periosteum; (2) stimulation of surrounding bone development walls off the area; (3) if the periosteum separates as a result of excess pressure, a sinus may develop, spreading the infection; and (4) possible spread of infection to involve the joint, causing infectious arthritis, and possible damage to the joint and epiphyseal plate.
9. Onset is more marked and large joints, such as knees, wrist, and elbows, are more frequently involved; more systemic effects are apparent.
10. Treatments for juvenile rheumatoid arthritis include: nonsteroidal antiinflammatory drugs and glucocorticoids if needed. Glucocorticoids may be required for severe inflammation or if organs such as the heart are affected. Disease-modifying antirheumatic drugs such as methotrexate may be used in small doses to slow the progress of the disease and prevent joint damage. Biologics can also be used to suppress the over action of the immune. system. Physiotherapy and exercise, particularly swimming, are important to maintain the flexibility, alignment, function, and proper development of the joints.
11. Anorexia nervosa is extreme weight loss due to self-starvation; bulimia is characterized by binge eating and purging.
12. *Propionibacterium acnes, Staphylococcus*
13. Epstein-Barr virus
14. Manifestations include sore throat, headache, fever, malaise, and fatigue; lymphadenopathy; rash on the trunk; lymphocytosis and monocytosis; and positive heterophil antibody. Complications include hepatitis, ruptured spleen, and meningitis.

Copyright © 2027 by Elsevier, Inc. All rights are reserved, including those for text and data mining, AI training, and similar technologies.

15. Turner syndrome: one X chromosome is missing. It affects sexual development in females and causes other abnormalities as well. Anomalies include malformations of the heart and genitourinary system, and retarded growth. At puberty, growth spurt, development of secondary sex characteristics, and initiation of menstrual cycle are absent.
16. the discomfort that occurs in varying degrees during the first or second day of menstruation

CHAPTER 24: Complications of Aging

1. genetically programmed (cell death [apoptosis]); "wear-and-tear" cellular damage; "free radicals" (*i.e.,* peroxides); other options: latent viruses, increased autoimmune reactions, environmental agents
2.
   i. In general, hormone secretions remain relatively constant, but tissue receptor sensitivity diminishes (see reproductive system for additional female changes, *i.e.,* menopause).
   ii. *female:* menopause, when ovaries cease production of estrogen and progesterone, resulting in rise in serum levels of follicle-stimulating hormone and luteinizing hormone; decreased sex hormone levels result in thinning of the mucosa, loss of elasticity and glandular secretions in the vagina and cervix, which may cause inflammation and dyspareunia; pH of vaginal secretions become more alkaline, predisposing to infections; breasts decrease in size; "hot flashes" due to hormone level changes; emotional lability
   male: gradual decline in testosterone, decrease in testes size and sperm production but remain potent or fertile; benign prostatic hypertrophy—common problem in older males
   iii. Both become thin and fragile; increased susceptibility to injury and inflammation; and slower wound healing.
   iv. Fatty tissue and collagen fibers accumulate in heart muscle; size and number of cardiac muscle cells decline, reducing strength of cardiac contractions. Pathological changes include vascular degeneration, which reduces cardiac output and reserve. Degenerative changes promote arteriosclerosis and atherosclerosis.
   v. Loss of calcium and bone mass due to aging may lead to osteoporosis, osteoarthritis, degeneration of intervertebral discs, and increased risk of herniation or rupture. Skeletal mass declines with aging, resulting in atrophy of skeletal muscle.
   vi. Ventilation decreases due to reduction of lung tissue elasticity; calcification of costal cartilage reduces movement; skeletal muscle atrophy; vascular degeneration leads to decreased perfusion and gas exchange.
   vii. Natural reduction in brain mass occurs with aging and leads to various degenerative changes in the brain; decline in various functions, including reflexes, memory, etc.; diminished autonomic nervous system adaptability, leading to temperature sensitivities; degenerative changes in the eye, resulting in various conditions such as presbyopia, cataracts, glaucoma; hearing loss; diminished sense of taste and smell—appetite loss.
   viii. increased risk of oral infections, periodontal disease, loss of teeth; decreased appetite, potential malnutrition; diminished salivation causes difficulty chewing and swallowing, xerostomia (dry mouth); swallowing difficulties due to medications or other neurological problems; obesity and associated disease risks (e.g., diabetes, gallstones, hypertension); atrophy of GI tract mucosa causing malabsorption of essential nutrients, including vitamins and minerals; predisposition to malignancy
   ix. reduced kidney function due to loss of glomeruli and degeneration of tubules; reduced bladder control—muscles become weaker as a result of aging
3. Infections are common as a result of impaired circulation and delayed or diminished healing capacity; diminished immune responsivity; urinary system disorders requiring frequent catheterization, predisposing to infection. Cancer is more common in the elderly—the immune system is less effective, and higher cumulative exposure to carcinogens has occurred.
4.
   a) inability to control urination; v. incontinence
   b) farsightedness; vii. presbyopia
   c) predetermined cell death; iii. apoptosis
   d) excessive urination at night; vi. nocturia
   e) opacity of the ocular lens; ii. cataract
   f) deposition of fat in arterial walls; i. atherosclerosis
   g) dry mouth; viii. xerostomia
   h) increased intraocular pressure; iv. glaucoma

CHAPTER 25: Immobility and Associated Problems

1. **musculoskeletal effects:** muscles lose strength, endurance, and mass very quickly, atrophy and develop flaccidity; impaired venous return, development of dependent edema; bone demineralization leading to osteoporosis, shortening and decreased flexibility of connective tissue such as ligaments and tendons
   cutaneous effects: impaired circulation leads to skin breakdown and reduced regeneration; decubitus ulcers
   cardiovascular effects: reduced venous return and cardiac output; orthostatic hypotension; blood pooling in dependent areas, resulting in edema; thrombus formation; potential embolism
   respiratory effects: decreased depth of respirations; diminished gaseous exchange; diminished cough resulting in fluid, secretion accumulation; predisposition to respiratory complications: infection, obstruction, and atelectasis; potential for food and water aspiration
   gastrointestinal effects: constipation; appetite reduction: malnutrition, fatigue, and depression
   urinary effects: urinary stasis with potential for calculus formation and urinary tract infection
   effects on children: normal growth delayed; spinal or bony deformities; other developmental disorders

Copyright © 2027 by Elsevier, Inc. All rights are reserved, including those for text and data mining, AI training, and similar technologies.

2.
   a) stationary blood clot; viii. thrombus
   b) collapse of lung tissue; i. atelectasis
   c) sudden drop in blood pressure when change in position occurs vi. orthostatic hypotension
   d) break away thrombus iv. embolus
   e) pressure sore or bedsore; iii. decubitus ulcer
   f) paralysis below the waist; vii. paraplegia
   g) joint deformity caused by excessive scarring; ii. contracture
   h) paralysis of one side of the body; v. hemiplegia
   i) loss of bone mass; x. osteoporosis
   j) loss of muscle tone; ix. flaccidity
3. sedatives (to promote sleep and reduce anxiety) and analgesics (to control pain)
4. Constipation is the major digestive system problem associated with immobility. Treatments include use of laxatives, increased intake of fluids and fiber, and in some cases treatment for GERD may be required.
5. Immobility may cause stasis of urine which can lead to kidney or bladder infections and the development of renal calculi.

CHAPTER 26: Stress and Associated Problems

1. A *stressor* is any factor that creates a significant change in the body's homeostasis. It may be physical, psychological, or both. Physical stressors: (1) Pain, causing increased heart rate; (2) Infection, initiating fever. Psychological stressors: (1) Anxiety, elevating cortisol levels; (2) New job, increasing mental arousal.
2. aging, pathological disorders
3. (Fig. 26.1) Norepinephrine from the sympathetic nervous system (SNS) and the adrenal medulla causes general vasoconstriction and increased blood pressure.
   Epinephrine from the adrenal medulla causes increased heart rate and general vasoconstriction, resulting in increased blood pressure, vasodilation in skeletal muscle, bronchodilation, and increased blood glucose.
   Adrenocorticotropic hormone (ACTH) from the anterior pituitary stimulates the adrenal cortex.
   Cortisol from the adrenal cortex results in increased stability in the cardiovascular system and enhances the effects of the catecholamines, elevates blood glucose, reduces inflammatory and immune responses, and stimulates the central nervous system (CNS).
   Aldosterone from the adrenal cortex increases the reabsorption of sodium and water, increasing blood pressure.
   Antidiuretic hormone from the posterior pituitary increases retention of water, increasing blood pressure.
4. (Fig. 26.1) Significant effects of the sympathetic nervous system during the stress response include elevated blood pressure and increased heart rate, bronchodilation and increased ventilation, increased blood glucose levels, and CNS arousal.
5. Prolonged stress can lead to a variety of serious complications, including disruption of intellectual function and memory, renal failure, or stress ulcers. Severe stress can also lead to infection due to depression of the inflammatory response and the immune system. Opportunistic infections may develop, and normally nonpathogenic organisms may cause infection. Continued stress may impede the healing of tissue following trauma or surgery. This may lead to increased risks for infection and scar tissue at the site.
6. adequate rest, healthy diet, change in lifestyle, regular moderate exercise, counseling and support services, relaxation techniques, antianxiety medications, assessing options/goals
7. Technostress refers to stress that is a result of the use of information and communication technologies (ICTs) and the expectations of ICT use in business and general society
8. (1) Alarm stage: Hypothalamus and sympathetic nervous system activate, increasing ACTH and adrenaline. (2) Resistance stage: Hormonal levels peak, optimizing body systems (e.g., increased glucose for energy). (3) Exhaustion stage: Body fails to cope, leading to damage (e.g., immune suppression) or systemic shutdown.

CHAPTER 27: Substance Abuse and Associated Problems

1. *physiological dependence*: the body has adapted to the drug so that discontinuing use will result in withdrawal signs such as tremors and/or cramps
   psychological dependence: a continuing desire to take the drug so as to function
   addiction: the uncontrollable compulsion to use the substance often, with serious consequences for the individual, the family, and society—considered the most serious form of substance abuse
2. psychological imbalances, personality deficits, biological abnormalities, dysfunctional interpersonal relationships, or some combination of any of these factors
3. first: lipid accumulation in the cells (fatty liver), second: inflammation and necrosis (alcoholic hepatitis), and third: fibrosis or scar tissue formation
4. for heroin addiction, methadone; for alcohol addiction, disulfiram (Antabuse)
5. Narcan (naloxone) is an opioid antagonistic drug used in treatment of opioid overdose.
6.
   a) Speed: iv. amphetamines
   b) Ecstasy: v. MDMA
   c) Blow: viii. heroin
   d) Angel dust: ii. phencyclidine
   e) Ice: i. methamphetamine
   f) Snow: vii. cocaine
   g) Special K: v. MDMA
   h) Weed: vi. Marijuana

Copyright © 2027 by Elsevier, Inc. All rights are reserved, including those for text and data mining, AI training, and similar technologies.

CHAPTER 28: Environmental Hazards and Associated Problems

1. damaging the cell membrane eventually causing cell lysis, alteration, or interference in cellular metabolic pathways, causing cellular mutations that could lead to cancer
2. hemolytic anemia, inflammation and/or ulceration of the digestive tract, inflammation of the kidney tubules, damage to the nervous system
3. particulate, an example is asbestos; gaseous, an example is sulfur dioxide
4. Hyperthermia is an excessive elevation of body temperature. Syndromes associated with it are heat cramps, heat exhaustion, and heat stroke.
5. Local hypothermia usually involves fingers, toes, ears, or exposed parts of the face and can result in necrosis/gangrene. Systemic hypothermia usually involves many body tissues over a wide area and can result in tissue necrosis as well as hypovolemic shock.
6. cells undergoing rapid mitosis such as epithelial tissue, bone marrow, and gonads
7. direct injection of toxin into body, transmission of an infectious agent through the bite/sting, allergic reaction to a substance in the bite/sting
8. (1) *E. coli*: Causes hemolytic uremic syndrome, damaging renal tubules and causing kidney failure. (2) *Shigella*: Causes dysentery with bloody diarrhea.
9. Excessive noise causes hearing loss by rupturing the tympanic membrane or damaging inner ear nerve cells, leading to tinnitus or irreversible hearing impairment. It may also cause stress-related effects like fatigue.

Copyright © 2027 by Elsevier, Inc. All rights are reserved,
including those for text and data mining, AI training, and similar technologies.